Acknowledgement

It gives us immense pleasure to thank Smt. S. S. Patil College of Pharmacy, Chopda, Maharashtra and Pacific University, Udaipur for their appreciation, moral support, constant encouragement, positive criticism and scientific inputs.

We are thankful to Prof. Dr. S. B. Bari, Dean of Pharmaceutical Science, North Maharashtra University, Jalgaon and Principal, H. R. Patel College of Pharmacy, Shirpur who encouraged us to pursue this attempt in all fronts. We thank our college staff and library staff who helped us at every step.

The authors are grateful to Prof. Dr. V. R. Patil, Principal, College of Pharmacy, Faizpur, India, Prof. Dr. Sunil P. Pawar, Chairman of Board of Studies, Department of Pharmacology & Pharmacognosy of North Maharashtra University, Jalgaon and Dr. G. P. Vadnere, Principal, Smt. S. S. Patil College of Pharmacy, Chopda, India for excellent guidance and dedicated efforts made us to think upon and understand number of problems and solve them judiciously.

Thankful to our colleagues and many users of the book for constructive criticism and suggestions.

We are grateful to our parents for their unconditional love, support and encouragement.

We are also thankful to my Publishers. We hope this book will leave the desired impression and look forward to receive any comments from the readers.

Authors

A Practical Book of

HUMAN ANATOMY AND PHYSIOLOGY - II

As Per PCI Regulations

FIRST YEAR B. PHARM.

Semester II

Dr. Md. Rageeb Md. Usman
M. Pharm., Ph.D., FAPP, FICPHS, FRSH, FSPER, FSRHCP
Joint Secretaries - SPER Central Branch &
President - IPA/APP/RSH/SRHCP
Maharashtra State Branch &
Associate Professor
Smt. S. S. Patil College of Pharmacy,
Chopda, Maharashtra
NMU Jalgaon, Maharashtra, India

Dr. Mrunal K. Shirsat
M. Pharm., Ph.D.
Principal and Professor
Pacific University
L.S.D.P. College of Pharmacy,
Mandvagan Pharata, Shirur
Pune.

Dr. Jayesh Dwivedi
M. Pharm., Ph.D.
Associate Professor
Pacific University
Pacific Academy of Higher Education and
Research University, Udaipur, Rajasthan
India

Dr. Mohammed Zuber Shaikh
M.Sc., Ph.D.
Head, Dept. of Zoology,
Senior Science College, Akkalkuwa, M.S., India

NIRALI PRAKASHAN ®
ADVANCEMENT OF KNOWLEDGE

N3942

Human Anatomy and Physiology - II (Practical) **ISBN 978-93-86943-50-7**

Fourth Edition : February 2020

Published By :

NIRALI PRAKASHAN

Abhyudaya Pragati, 1312, Shivaji Nagar,
Off J.M. Road, PUNE – 411005
Tel - (020) 25512336/37/39, Fax - (020) 25511379
Email : niralipune@pragationline.com

➢ DISTRIBUTION CENTRES

PUNE

Nirali Prakashan (For orders within Pune) : 119, Budhwar Peth, Jogeshwari Mandir Lane, Pune 411002, Maharashtra
Tel : (020) 2445 2044, Mobile : 9657703145
Email : niralilocal@pragationline.com

Nirali Prakashan (For orders outside Pune) : S. No. 28/27, Dhayari, Near Asian College Pune 411041
Tel : (020) 24690204 Fax : (020) 24690316; Mobile : 9657703143
Email : bookorder@pragationline.com

MUMBAI

Nirali Prakashan : 385, S.V.P. Road, Rasdhara Co-op. Hsg. Society Ltd.,
Girgaum, Mumbai 400004, Maharashtra; Mobile : 9320129587
Tel : (022) 2385 6339 / 2386 9976, Fax : (022) 2386 9976
Email : niralimumbai@pragationline.com

➢ DISTRIBUTION BRANCHES

JALGAON

Nirali Prakashan : 34, V. V. Golani Market, Navi Peth, Jalgaon 425001, Maharashtra,
Tel : (0257) 222 0395, Mob : 94234 91860; Email : niralijalgaon@pragationline.com

KOLHAPUR

Nirali Prakashan : New Mahadvar Road, Kedar Plaza, 1st Floor Opp. IDBI Bank, Kolhapur 416 012
Maharashtra. Mob : 9850046155; Email : niralikolhapur@pragationline.com

NAGPUR

Nirali Prakashan : Above Maratha Mandir, Shop No. 3, First Floor,
Rani Jhanshi Square, Sitabuldi, Nagpur 440012, Maharashtra
Tel : (0712) 254 7129; Email : niralinagpur@pragationline.com

DELHI

Nirali Prakashan : 4593/15, Basement, Agarwal Lane, Ansari Road, Daryaganj
Near Times of India Building, New Delhi 110002 Mob : 08505972553
Email : niralidelhi@pragationline.com

BENGALURU

Nirali Prakashan : Maitri Ground Floor, Jaya Apartments, No. 99, 6th Cross, 6th Main,
Malleswaram, Bengaluru 560003, Karnataka; Mob : 9449043034
Email: niralibangalore@pragationline.com

Other Branches : Hyderabad, Chennai

niralipune@pragationline.com | www.pragationline.com

Also find us on www.facebook.com/niralibooks

Preface

This book with the title "A Practical Book of Human Anatomy and Physiology - II" is written with an intention to benefit the Diploma and Degree students.

Practical aspect of Human Anatomy and Physiology serves as an essential study feature of Diploma and Degree Pharmacy Course which enrich the knowledge of the student pharmacists and makes the Pharmacist easy to understand drug action and technology of drug dosage form.

The book of Human Anatomy and Physiology - II has been specifically designed as per PCI New Syllabus for First Year B. Pharmacy Students.

Pharmacy Council of India are Prescribed by New Syllabus of all over India.

The matter is precise, appropriate and with easy to understand language. The accurate and clear diagrams provide a better approach towards understanding the features.

Any valuable and useful suggestions for the improvement of this book are always welcomed.

Hope this will be helpful....All the best!!!

Authors

Syllabus

1. To study the integumentary and special senses using specimen, models, etc.
2. To study the nervous system using specimen, models, etc.
3. To study the endocrine system using specimen, models, etc.
4. To demonstrate the general neurological examination
5. To demonstrate the function of olfactory nerve
6. To examine the different types of taste.
7. To demonstrate the visual acuity
8. To demonstrate the reflex activity
9. Recording of body temperature
10. To demonstrate positive and negative feedback mechanism.
11. Determination of tidal volume and vital capacity.
12. Study of digestive, respiratory, cardiovascular systems, urinary and reproductive systems with the help of models, charts and specimens.
13. Recording of basal mass index.
14. Study of family planning devices and pregnancy diagnosis test.
15. Demonstration of total blood count by cell analyser.
16. Permanent slides of vital organs and gonads.

***

Contents

***

Experiment No. 01

Aim: To study the compound microscope.

Microscope:

A microscope (from the Ancient Greek: *mikros*, "small" and *skopein*, "to look" or "see") is an instrument used to see objects that are too small for the naked eye. The science of investigating small object using such an instrument is called microscopy. Microscopic means invisible to the eye unless aided by a microscope. There are many types of microscopes, the most common and first to be invented is the optical microscope which uses light to image the sample. Other major types of microscopes are the electron microscope (both the transmission electron microscope and the scanning electron microscope) and the various types of scanning probe microscope.

Zacharias Jansen invented first compound microscope. When the microscope was invented around 1590, suddenly we saw a new world of living things in our water, in our food and under our nose. But it's unclear who invented the microscope. Some historians say it was **Hans Lippershey**, most famous for filing the first patent for a telescope.

Types of Microscope:

1. Simple microscope
2. Compound microscope
3. Electronic microscope
4. Motic microscope

1. Simple Microscope:

A simple microscope is a microscope which has only one lens, as opposed to the compound lenses used in more complex microscope designs. Magnifying glasses and loupes are two well-known examples of the simple microscope. The image quality with a simple microscope can be surprisingly good, as researchers learned when they used replications of 17th century simple microscopes to see what exactly it was that biologists found in water supplies in the early days of microscopy. If the lens is of a very high quality, the user should know how to manipulate the microscope to achieve the best focus, contrast and clarity. The image can be quite excellent, although it is of course impossible to obtain very high levels of magnification with a simple microscope. For basic applications, however, this design can be quite useful, in addition to affordable for people who may not want to shell out for a more advanced microscope design.

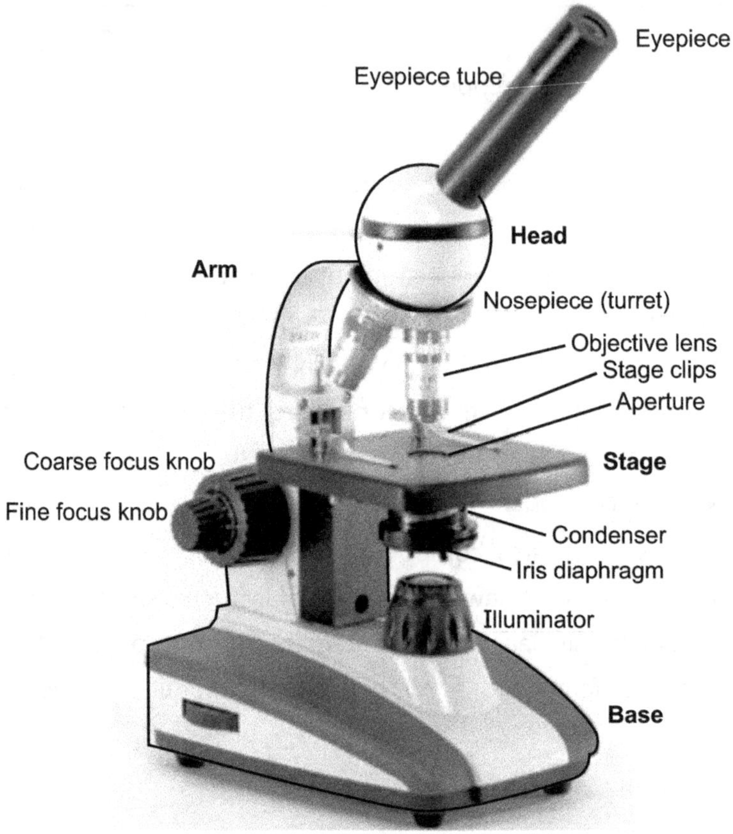

Fig. 1.1: Simple Microscope

2. Compound Microscope:

A **compound microscope** is a microscope with more than one lens and its own light source. In this type of microscope, there are ocular lenses in the binocular eyepieces and objective lenses in a rotating nosepiece closer to the specimen. Although sometimes found as monocular with one ocular lens and the compound binocular microscope is more commonly used today. They combine the power of lenses and light to enlarge the subject being viewed.

Viewing Heads: Monocular, Binocular, Trinocular:

- **Monocular:** Monocular only use one eyepiece when viewing the specimen. You are restricted if you want to use a CCD camera because this would occupy the eyepiece. However, monocular microscopes are light weight and are inexpensive.
- **Binocular:** They have two eyepieces which prove to be more comfortable. It is the most common choice.
- **Trinocular:** Trinocular has a third eyepiece tube that can be used by another person simultaneously or by a CCD camera. The trinocular option is more expensive than the other two types.

Typically, the eyepiece itself allows for 10X or 15X magnifications and when combined with the three or four objective lenses which can be rotated into the field of view. They produce higher magnification to a maximum of around 1000X generally. The compound light microscope is popular among botanists for studying plant cells in biology to view bacteria and parasites as well as a variety of human/animal cells.

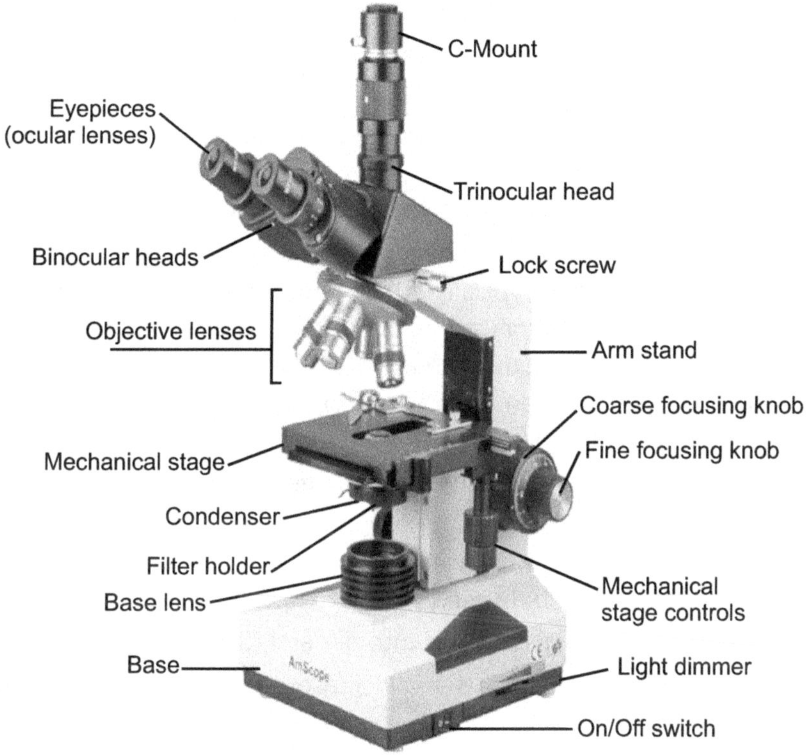

Fig. 1.2: Compound Microscope

The compound microscope essentially consists of three major systems.

1. **Support system:**

   It comprises of base, stage and body tube.

   Base: The base supports the microscope and it's where illuminator is located.

   Stage: The flat platform where the slide is placed. The specimen is the object being examined. Most specimens are mounted on slides, flat rectangles of thin glass. The specimen is placed on the glass and a cover slip is placed over the specimen. This allows the slide to be easily inserted or removed from the microscope. It also allows the specimen to be labeled, transported, and stored without damage.

   Stage clips: Metal clips that hold the slide in place.

   Stage height adjustment (Stage Control): These knobs move the stage left and right or up and down.

   Body tube (Head): The body tube connects the eyepiece to the objective lenses. The arm connects the body tube to the base of the microscope.

2. **Illumination system:**

It comprises of light source or mirror, iris diaphragm and condenser. It is the light source for a microscope. Older microscopes used mirrors to reflect light from an external source up through the bottom of the stage; however, most microscopes now use a low-voltage bulb. The switch on the base of the microscope turns the illuminator off and on

Iris diaphragm: Adjusts the amount of light that reaches the specimen.

Condenser: Gathers and focuses light from the illuminator onto the specimen being viewed.

3. **Magnification system:**

This includes objective (is a set of lenses placed near the object, it partially magnifies the object) and eyepiece (a more magnified form of real image is observed). Compound microscope, take the power of the objective lens which is at 4X, 10X or 45X and multiply it by the power of the eyepiece which is typically 10X. Therefore, a 10X eyepiece used with a 45X objective lens will produce a magnification of 400X. The naked eye can now view the specimen at a magnification 400 times greater and so microscopic details are revealed. Magnification is the ability to view an object as larger. A good image is obtained when the amount of specimen detail is also increased.

Eyepiece: The lens the viewer looks through to see the specimen. The eyepiece usually contains a 10X or 15X power lens.

Diopter Adjustment: Useful as a means to change focus on one eyepiece so as to correct for any difference in vision between your two eyes.

Coarse adjustment: Brings the specimen into general focus.

Fine adjustment: Fine tunes the focus and increases the detail of the specimen.

Nosepiece: A rotating turret that houses the objective lenses. The viewer spins the nosepiece to select different objective lenses.

Objective lenses: One of the most important parts of a compound microscope, as they are the lenses closest to the specimen. A standard microscope has three, four, or five objective lenses that range in power from 4X to 100X. When focusing the microscope, be careful that the objective lens doesn't touch the slide, as it could break the slide and destroy the specimen.

Uses of Compound Microscope:

One of the biggest benefits of owning a light microscope is its simplicity and its convenience. A compound light microscope is relatively small, therefore it's easy to use and simple to store and it comes with its own light source. Moreover, because of their multiple lenses the compound light microscopes are able to reveal a great amount of detail in samples. Even an inexpensive one can reveal an incredible view of the world that would be impossible to explore with the naked eye.

Instructions:

1. Always use the microscope in vertical direction.
2. Do not make the use of direct sunlight.

3. The object to be examined should be mounted in mounting medium & should be covered with cover slip before observation.

Precautions:

1. Do not keep the microscope near the edge of the table.
2. Always keep the stage clean and dry.
3. Do not use excess mounting medium.
4. Microscope when not in use should be covered properly.

3. Electronic Microscope:

An EM is a microscope that focuses beams of energetic electrons to examine objects up to nano-scales. They utilize the same principles behind an optical microscope, but rather than photons or particles of light, concentrate electrons, charged particles located on the outside of atoms, onto an object. Additional differences include preparation of specimens before being placed in the vacuum chamber, the use of coiled electromagnets instead of glass lenses, the use of a thermionic gun as an electron source and the image or electron micrograph is viewed on a screen rather than an eyepiece. All EMs use electromagnetic or electrostatic lenses, which consist of a coil of wire wrapped around the outside of a tube, commonly referred to as a solenoid.

In addition, EMs use digital displays, computer interfaces, software for image analysis and a low vacuum or variable pressure chamber, which upholds the pressure differential between the high vacuum levels essential to the gun and column area and the low pressure required in the chamber.

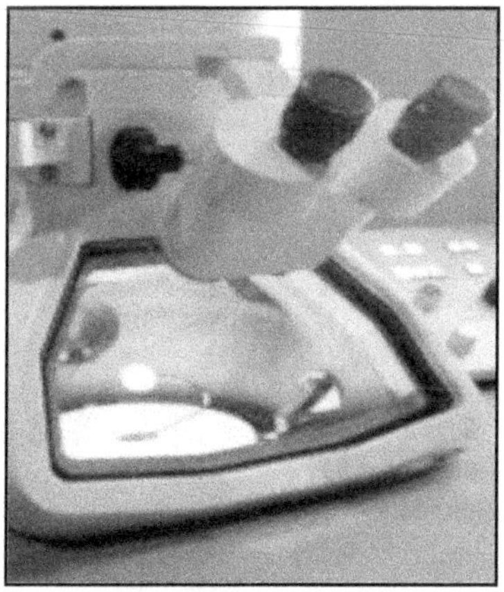

Fig. 1.3: Electronic Microscope

All electron microscopy samples must be prepared before placed in the microscope vacuum. Techniques, which vary based on type of specimen and analysis, include:

- Cryofixation
- Fixation
- Dehydration

- Embedding
- Sectioning
- Staining
- Freeze-fracture and Freeze-etch
- Sputter Coating

Most of these techniques require specialized training and, due to sample manipulation, can result in artifacts or inadvertent changes to the structure of the specimen.

The following gives you a description of two types of EMs, the Transmission (TEM) and Scanning Electron Microscope (SEM).

Transmission Electron Microscope:

The transmission electron microscope (TEM), the first type of EM, has many commonalities with the optical microscope and is a powerful microscope, capable of producing images 1 nanometer in size. They require high voltages to increase the acceleration speed of electrons, which, once they pass through the sample (transmission), increase the image resolution. The 2-d, black and white images produced by TEMs can be seen on a screen or printed onto a photographic plate. Although recent innovations in software help to minimize, TEM resolution is hampered by spherical and chromatic aberrations. The TEM is a popular choice for nanotechnology as well as semiconductor analysis and production.

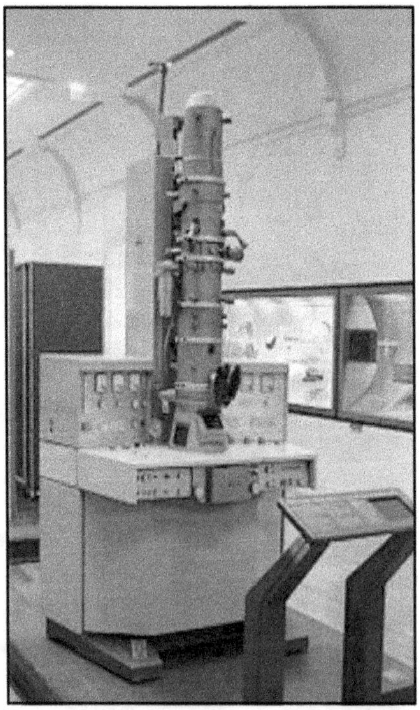

Fig. 1.4: Transmission Electron Microscope

Scanning Electron Microscope:

Reflecting light microscopes are the optical counterpart to scanning electron microscopes (SEM) and produce similar data. SEMs are primarily used to obtain topographical information. In this type of EM, a series of solenoids pulls the beam back and forth across the sample, systematically scanning the surface; it detects secondary electrons emitted from the surface and produces an image. Although SEMs are approximately 10 times less powerful than TEMs, they produce high-resolution, sharp, black and white 3D images

4. Motic Microscope:

Motic is one of the first microscope manufacturers who started to develop digital microscopy solutions, digital imaging products and application software. This new development in microscopy has lead to a complete range of digital microscopes, digital cameras and software for all types of applications.

Motic Microscopes are highly regarded for their quality, innovative and extensive line of microscopes and digital cameras for the educational, medical, research, scientific and industrial markets worldwide.

The range includes CMOS and CCD cameras with different chip sizes and resolution. All digital microscopes and Moticam cameras come as an all-in-one-box concept that includes software, calibration slide, eyepiece adapters with the cameras and much more.

This microscope add on can produce images in high resolution that can be viewed on any LCD screens and is an excellent tool for any life science, medical and education field.

New York Microscope Company is the only microscope company to offer Free Service Protection Guarantee with the purchase of every microscope.

The importance of documentation has expanded into every aspect of microscopy, as has the method of documentation.

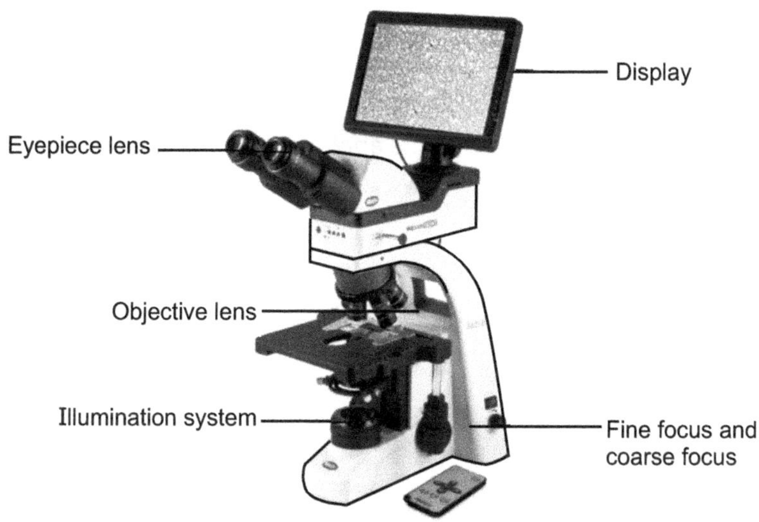

Fig. 1.5: Motic Microscope with Printer

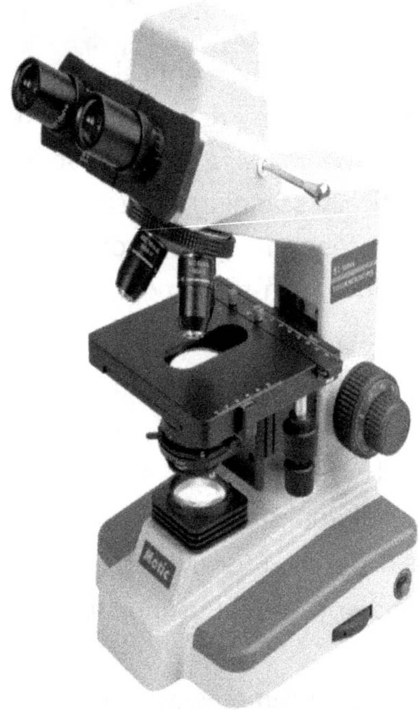

Fig. 1.6: Motic Microscope

Result:

Questions

1. What are different types of microscopes?
2. Write the use of each type of microscope.
3. Who invented the first microscope?
4. Who invented compound microscope?
5. Define magnification value of microscope.
6. What is electron microscope? Write its applications.

***

Experiment No. 02

Aim: To study the integumentary and special senses system using specimen, models etc.

Requirements:

1. Model of integumentary system.
2. Charts of integumentary system.
3. Specimen of integumentary system.

Theory:

The integumentary system is an organ system consisting of the skin, hair, nails, and exocrine glands. The skin is only a few millimeters thick yet is by far the largest organ in the body. The average person's skin weighs 10 pounds and has a surface area of almost 20 square feet. Skin forms the body's outer covering and forms a barrier to protect the body from chemicals, disease, UV light, and physical damage. Hair and nails extend from the skin to reinforce the skin and protect it from environmental damage. The exocrine glands of the integumentary system produce sweat, oil, and wax to cool, protect, and moisturize the skin's surface.

Functions of the Integumentary System:

The integumentary system has many functions, most of which are involved in protecting the body and regulating body's internal functions in a variety of ways:

- Protects the body's internal living tissues and organs.
- Protects against invasion by infectious organisms.
- Protects the body from dehydration.
- Protects the body against abrupt changes in temperature.
- Helps dispose of waste materials.
- Acts as a receptor for touch, pressure, pain, heat, and cold.
- Stores water and fat.

How does the integumentary system work with other systems?

The body is a complicated system that consists of many subsystems that help to keep it functioning properly. These subsystems serve a variety of purposes and require needed materials to function properly, as well as means of communicating information to other parts of the body. Thus, the skin and other parts of the integumentary system work with other systems in our body to maintain and support the conditions that your cells, tissues, and organs need to function properly.

The skin is one of the first defense mechanisms in our immune system. Tiny glands in the skin secrete oils that enhance the barrier function of the skin. Immune cells live in the skin and provide the first line of defense against infections.

By helping to synthesize and absorb vitamin D, the integumentary system works with the digestive system to encourage the uptake of calcium from our diet. This substance enters the blood stream though the capillary networks in the skin. Healthy functioning of the skin is also related to the digestive system because the digestion and assimilation of dietary fats and oils are essential for the body to be able to make the protective oils for the skin and hair.

The integumentary system also works closely with the circulatory system and the surface capillaries through our body. Because certain substances can enter the blood stream through the capillary networks in the skin, patches can be used to deliver medications in this manner for conditions ranging from heart problems (nitroglycerin) to smoking cessation (nicotine patches).

The skin is also important in helping to regulate our body temperature. If you are too hot or too cold, your brain sends nerve impulses to the skin, which has three ways to either increase or decrease heat loss from the body's surface: hairs on the skin trap more warmth if they are standing up, and less if they are lying flat; glands under the skin secrete sweat on to the surface of the skin in order to increase heat loss by evaporation if the body is too hot; capillaries near the surface can open when the body needs to cool off and close when the need to conserve heat.

The skin plays a vital role in the body as regards the sense of touch. The nervous system depends on neurons embedded in your skin to sense the outside world. It processes input from the senses, including touch, and initiates actions based on those inputs. For example, when you stub your toe, nerve cells in the foot send signals up the leg, through the spinal cord, and up into the brain. The nerve cell connections in the brain sense these signals as pain.

As well as interacting with the body systems as explained above, the integumentary system also contributes to numerous physiological processes, especially those involved in the regulation of the body's internal environment so as to maintain a stable condition. An example is provided by the way that the skin helps in temperature regulation by changes in the pattern of blood supply to the skin and by sweating, as mentioned above.

Epidermis:

The epidermis is the most superficial layer of the skin that covers almost the entire body surface. The epidermis rests upon and protects the deeper and thicker dermis layer of the skin. Structurally, the epidermis is only about a tenth of a millimeter thick but is made of 40 to 50 rows of stacked squamous epithelial cells. The epidermis is an avascular region of the body, meaning that it does not contain any blood or blood vessels. The cells of the epidermis receive all of their nutrients via diffusion of fluids from the dermis.

The epidermis is made of several specialized types of cells. Almost 90% of the epidermis is made of cells known as keratinocytes. Keratinocytes develop from stem cells at the base of the epidermis and begin to produce and store the protein keratin. Keratin makes the keratinocytes very tough, scaly and water-resistant. At about 8% of epidermal cells, melanocytes form the second most numerous cell type in the epidermis. Melanocytes produce the pigment melanin to protect the skin from ultraviolet radiation and sunburn. Langerhans cells are the third most common cells in the epidermis and make up just over 1% of all epidermal cells. Langerhans cells' role is to detect and fight pathogens that attempt to enter the body through the skin. Finally, Merkel cells make up less than 1% of all epidermal cells but have the important function of sensing touch. Merkel cells form a disk along the deepest edge of the epidermis where they connect to nerve endings in the dermis to sense light touch.

The epidermis in most of the body is arranged into 4 distinct layers. In the palmar surface of the hands and plantar surface of the feet, the skin is thicker than in the rest of the body and there is a fifth layer of epidermis. The deepest region of the epidermis is the stratum basale, which contains the stem cells that reproduce to form all of the other cells of the epidermis. The cells of the stratum basale include cuboidal keratinocytes, melanocytes, and Merkel cells. Superficial to stratum basale is the stratum spinosum layer where Langerhans cells are found along with many rows of spiny keratinocytes. The spines found here are cellular projections called desmosomes that form between keratinocytes to hold them together and resist friction. Just superficial to the stratum spinosum is the stratum granulosum, where keratinocytes begin to produce waxy lamellar granules to waterproof the skin. The keratinocytes in the stratum granulosum are so far removed from the dermis that they begin to die from lack of nutrients. In the thick skin of the hands and feet, there is a layer of skin superficial to the stratum granulosum known as the stratum lucidum. The stratum lucidum is made of several rows of clear, dead keratinocytes that protect the underlying layers. The outermost layer of skin is the stratum corneum. The stratum corneum is made of many rows of flattened, dead keratinocytes that protect the underlying layers. Dead keratinocytes are constantly being shed from the surface of the stratum corneum and being replaced by cells arriving from the deeper layers.

Dermis:

The dermis is the deep layer of the skin found under the epidermis. The dermis is mostly made of dense irregular connective tissue along with nervous tissue, blood, and blood vessels. The dermis is much thicker than the epidermis and gives the skin its strength and elasticity. Within the dermis there are two distinct regions: the papillary layer and the reticular layer.

The papillary layer is the superficial layer of the dermis that borders on the epidermis. The papillary layer contains many finger-like extensions called dermal papillae that protrude superficially towards the epidermis. The dermal papillae increase the surface area of the dermis and contain many nerves and blood vessels that are projected toward the surface of the skin. Blood flowing through the dermal papillae provide nutrients and oxygen for the cells of the epidermis. The nerves of the dermal papillae are used to feel touch, pain, and temperature through the cells of the epidermis.

The deeper layer of the dermis, the reticular layer, is the thicker and tougher part of the dermis. The reticular layer is made of dense irregular connective tissue that contains many tough collagen and stretchy elastin fibers running in all directions to provide strength and elasticity to the skin. The reticular layer also contains blood vessels to support the skin cells and nerve tissue to sense pressure and pain in the skin.

Hypodermis:

Deep to the dermis is a layer of loose connective tissues known as the hypodermis, subcutis, or subcutaneous tissue. The hypodermis serves as the flexible connection between the skin and the underlying muscles and bones as well as a fat storage area. Areolar connective tissue in the hypodermis contains elastin and collagen fibers loosely arranged to allow the skin to stretch and move independently of its underlying structures. Fatty adipose tissue in the hypodermis stores energy in the form of triglycerides. Adipose also helps to insulate the body by trapping body heat produced by the underlying muscles.

Hair:

Hair is an accessory organ of the skin made of columns of tightly packed dead keratinocytes found in most regions of the body. The few hairless parts of the body include the palmar surface of the hands, plantar surface of the feet, lips, labia minora, and glans penis. Hair helps to protect the body from UV radiation by preventing sunlight from striking the skin. Hair also insulates the body by trapping warm air around the skin.

The structure of hair can be broken down into 3 major parts: the follicle, root, and shaft. The hair follicle is a depression of epidermal cells deep into the dermis. Stem cells in the follicle reproduce to form the keratinocytes that eventually form the hair while melanocytes produce pigment that gives the hair its colour. Within the follicle is the hair root, the portion of the hair below the skin's surface. As the follicle produces new hair, the cells in the root push up to the surface until they exit the skin. The hair shaft consists of the part of the hair that is found outside of the skin.

The hair shaft and root are made of 3 distinct layers of cells: the cuticle, cortex, and medulla. The cuticle is the outermost layer made of keratinocytes. The keratinocytes of the cuticle are stacked on top of each other like shingles so that the outer tip of each cell points away from the body. Under the cuticle are the cells of the cortex that form the majority of the hair's width. The spindle-shaped and tightly packed cortex cells contain pigments that give the hair its colour. The innermost layer of the hair, the medulla, is not present in all hairs. When present, the medulla usually contains highly pigmented cells full of keratin. When the medulla is absent, the cortex continues through the middle of the hair.

Nails:

Nails are accessory organs of the skin made of sheets of hardened keratinocytes and found on the distal ends of the fingers and toes. Fingernails and toenails reinforce and protect the end of the digits and are used for scraping and manipulating small aims. There are 3 main parts of a nail: the root, body, and free edge. The nail root is the portion of the nail found under the surface of the skin. The nail body is the visible external portion of the nail. The free edge is the distal end portion of the nail that has grown beyond the end of the finger or toe.

Nails grow from a deep layer of epidermal tissue known as the nail matrix, which surrounds the nail root. The stem cells of the nail matrix reproduce to form keratinocytes, which in turn produce keratin protein and pack into tough sheets of hardened cells. The sheets of keratinocytes form the hard nail root that slowly grows out of the skin and forms the nail body as it reaches the skin's surface. The cells of the nail root and nail body are pushed toward the distal end of the finger or toe by new cells being formed in the nail matrix. Under the nail body is a layer of epidermis and dermis known as the nail bed. The nail bed is pink in colour due to the presence of capillaries that support the cells of the nail body. The proximal end of the nail near the root forms a whitish crescent shape known as the lunula where a small amount of nail matrix is visible through the nail body. Around the proximal and lateral edges of the nail is the eponychium, a layer of epithelium that overlaps and covers the edge of the nail body. The eponychium helps to seal the edges of the nail to prevent infection of the underlying tissues.

Sudoriferous Glands:

Sudoriferous glands are exocrine glands found in the dermis of the skin and commonly known as sweat glands. There are 2 major types of sudoriferous glands: eccrine sweat glands and apocrine sweat glands. Eccrine sweat glands are found in almost every region of the skin and produce a secretion of water and sodium chloride. Eccrine sweat is delivered via a duct to the surface of the skin and is used to lower the body's temperature through evaporative cooling.

Apocrine sweat glands are found mainly the axillary and pubic regions of the body. The ducts of apocrine sweat glands extend into the follicles of hairs so that the sweat produced by these glands exits the body along the surface of the hair shaft. Apocrine sweat glands are inactive until puberty, at which point they produce a thick, oily liquid that is consumed by bacteria living on the skin. The digestion of apocrine sweat by bacteria produces body odour.

Sebaceous Glands:

Sebaceous glands are exocrine glands found in the dermis of the skin that produce an oily secretion known as sebum. Sebaceous glands are found in every part of the skin except for the thick skin of the palms of the hands and soles of the feet. Sebum is produced in the sebaceous glands and carried through ducts to the surface of the skin or to hair follicles. Sebum acts to waterproof and increase the elasticity of the skin. Sebum also lubricates and protects the cuticles of hairs as they pass through the follicles to the exterior of the body.

Ceruminous Glands:

Ceruminous glands are special exocrine glands found only in the dermis of the ear canals. Ceruminous glands produce a waxy secretion known as cerumen to protect the ear canals and lubricate the eardrum. Cerumen protects the ears by trapping foreign material such as dust and airborne pathogens that enter the ear canal. Cerumen is made continuously and slowly pushes older cerumen outward toward the exterior of the ear canal where it falls out of the ear or is manually removed.

Keratinization:

Keratinization, also known as cornification, is the process of keratin accumulating within keratinocytes. Keratinocytes begin their life as offspring of the stem cells of the stratum basale. Young keratinocytes have a cuboidal shape and contain almost no keratin protein at all. As the stem cells multiply, they push older keratinocytes towards the surface of the skin and into the superficial layers of the epidermis. By the time keratinocytes reach the stratum spinosum, they have begun to accumulate a significant amount of keratin and have become harder, flatter, and more water resistant. As the keratinocytes reach the stratum granulosum, they have become much flatter and are almost completely filled with keratin. At this point the cells are so far removed from the nutrients that diffuse from the blood vessels in the dermis that the cells go through the process of apoptosis. Apoptosis is programmed cell death where the cell digests its own nucleus and organelles, leaving only a tough, keratin-filled shell behind. Dead keratinocytes moving into the stratum lucidum and stratum corneum are very flat, hard, and tightly packed so as to form a keratin barrier to protect the underlying tissues.

Temperature Homeostasis:

Being the body's outermost organ, the skin is able to regulate the body temperature by controlling how the body interacts with its environment. In the case of the body entering a state of hyperthermia, the skin is able to reduce body temperature through sweating and vasodilation. Sweat produced by sudoriferous glands delivers water to the surface of the body where it begins to evaporate. The evaporation of sweat absorbs heat and cools the body's surface. Vasodilation is the process through which smooth muscle lining the blood vessels in the dermis relax and allow more blood to enter the skin. Blood transports heat through the body, pulling heat away from the body's core and depositing it in the skin where it can radiate out of the body and into the external environment.

In the case of the body entering a state of hypothermia, the skin is able to raise body temperature through the contraction of arrector pili muscles and through vasoconstriction. The follicles of hairs have small bundles of smooth muscle attached to their base called arrector pili muscles. The arrector pili form goose bumps by contracting to move the hair follicle and lifting the hair shaft upright from the surface of the skin. This movement results in more air being trapped under the hairs to insulate the surface of the body. Vasoconstriction is the process of smooth muscles in the walls of blood vessels in the dermis contracting to reduce the flow of blood to the skin. Vasoconstriction permits the skin to cool while blood stays in the body's core to maintain heat and circulation in the vital organs.

Vitamin D Synthesis:

Vitamin D, an essential vitamin necessary for the absorption of calcium from food, is produced by ultraviolet (UV) light striking the skin. The stratum basale and stratum spinosum layers of the epidermis contain a sterol molecule known as 7-dehydrocholesterol. When UV light present in sunlight or tanning bed lights strikes the skin, it penetrates through the outer layers of the epidermis and strikes some of the molecules of 7-dehydrocholesterol, converting it into vitamin D3. Vitamin D3 is converted in the kidneys into calcitriol, the active form of vitamin D.

Protection:

The skin provides protection to its underlying tissues from pathogens, mechanical damage, and UV light. Pathogens, such as viruses and bacteria, are unable to enter the body through unbroken skin due to the outermost layers of epidermis containing an unending supply of tough, dead keratinocytes. This protection explains the necessity of cleaning and covering cuts and scrapes with bandages to prevent infection. Minor mechanical damage from rough or sharp object is mostly absorbed by the skin before it can damage the underlying tissues. Epidermal cells reproduce constantly to quickly repair any damage to the skin. Melanocytes in the epidermis produce the pigment melanin, which absorbs UV light before it can pass through the skin. UV light can cause cells to become cancerous if not blocked from entering the body.

Skin Colour:

Human skin colour is controlled by the interaction of 3 pigments: melanin, carotene, and hemoglobin. Melanin is a brown or black pigment produced by melanocytes to protect the skin from UV radiation. Melanin gives skin its tan or brown colouration and provides the colour of brown or black hair. Melanin production increases as the skin is exposed to higher levels of UV light resulting in tanning of the skin. Carotene is another pigment present in the skin that produces a yellow or orange cast to the skin and is most noticeable in people with low levels of melanin. Haemoglobin is another pigment most noticeable in people with little melanin. Haemoglobin is the red pigment found in red blood cells, but can be seen through the layers of the skin as a light red or pink colour. Haemoglobin is most noticeable in skin colouration during times of vasodilation when the capillaries of the dermis are open to carry more blood to the skin's surface.

Cutaneous Sensation:

The skin allows the body to sense its external environment by picking up signals for touch, pressure, vibration, temperature, and pain. Merkel disks in the epidermis connect to nerve cells in the dermis to detect shapes and textures of object contacting the skin. Corpuscles of touch are structures found in the dermal papillae of the dermis that also detect touch by Aims contacting the skin. Lamellar corpuscles found deep in the dermis sense pressure and vibration of the skin. Throughout the dermis there are many free nerve endings that are simply neurons with their dendrites spread throughout the dermis. Free nerve endings may be sensitive to pain, warmth, or cold. The density of these sensory receptors in the skin varies throughout the body, resulting in some regions of the body being more sensitive to touch, temperature, or pain than other regions.

Excretion:

In addition to secreting sweat to cool the body, eccrine sudoriferous glands of the skin also excrete waste products out of the body. Sweat produced by eccrine sudoriferous glands normally contains mostly water with many electrolytes and a few other trace chemicals. The most common electrolytes found in sweat are sodium and chloride, but potassium, calcium, and magnesium ions may be excreted as well. When these electrolytes reach high levels in the blood, their presence in sweat also increases, helping to reduce their presence within the body. In addition to electrolytes, sweat contains and helps to excrete small amounts of metabolic waste products such as lactic acid, urea, uric acid, and ammonia. Finally, eccrine sudoriferous glands help to excrete alcohol from the body of someone who has been drinking alcoholic beverages. Alcohol causes vasodilation in the dermis, leading to increased perspiration as more blood reaches sweat glands. The alcohol in the blood is absorbed by the cells of the sweat glands, causing it to be excreted along with the other components of sweat.

Result:

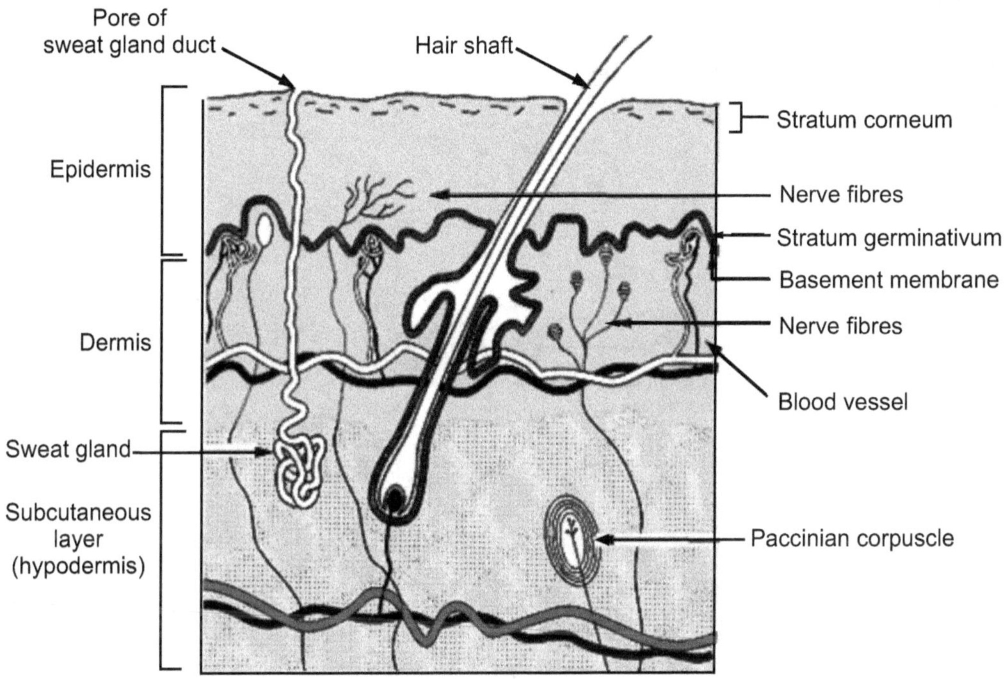

Fig. 2.1: Integumentary System

Questions

1. How do the integumentary system and the immune system work together?
2. What are the major organs of the integumentary system?
3. Why is the integumentary system important?
4. How many layers does the integumentary system have?

***

Experiment No. 03

Aim: To study the structure and functions of central nervous system using specimen and models etc.

Requirements:

1. Model of central nervous system.
2. Chart of central nervous system.

Theory:

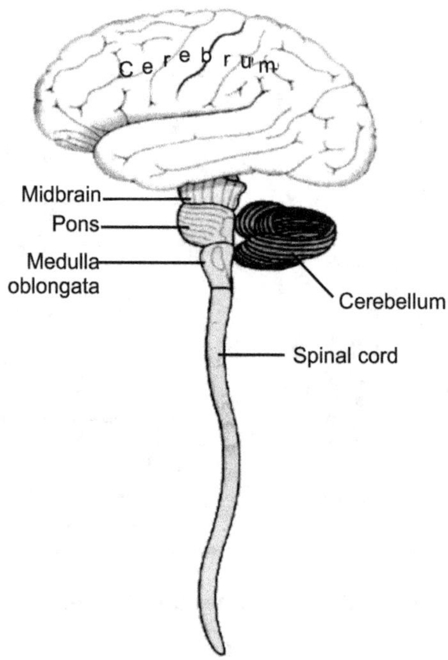

Fig. 3.1: Structure of Brain

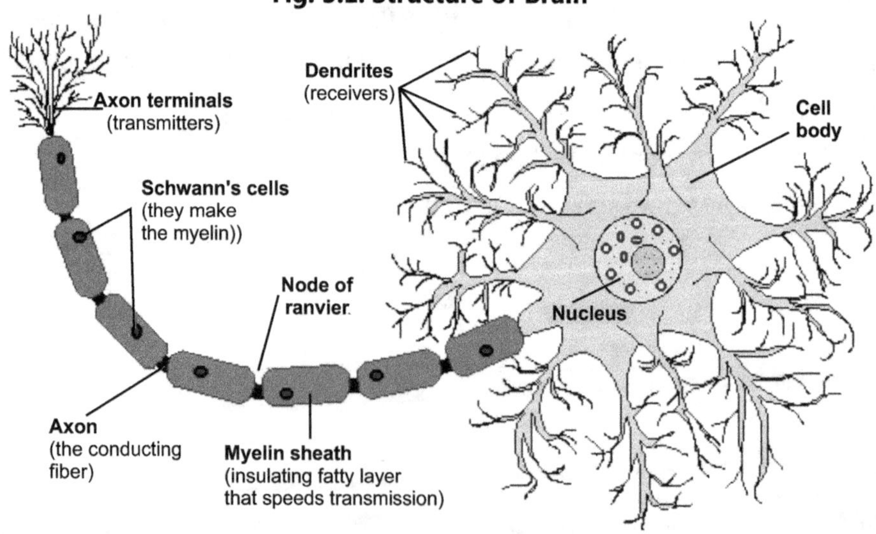

Fig. 3.2: Neuron

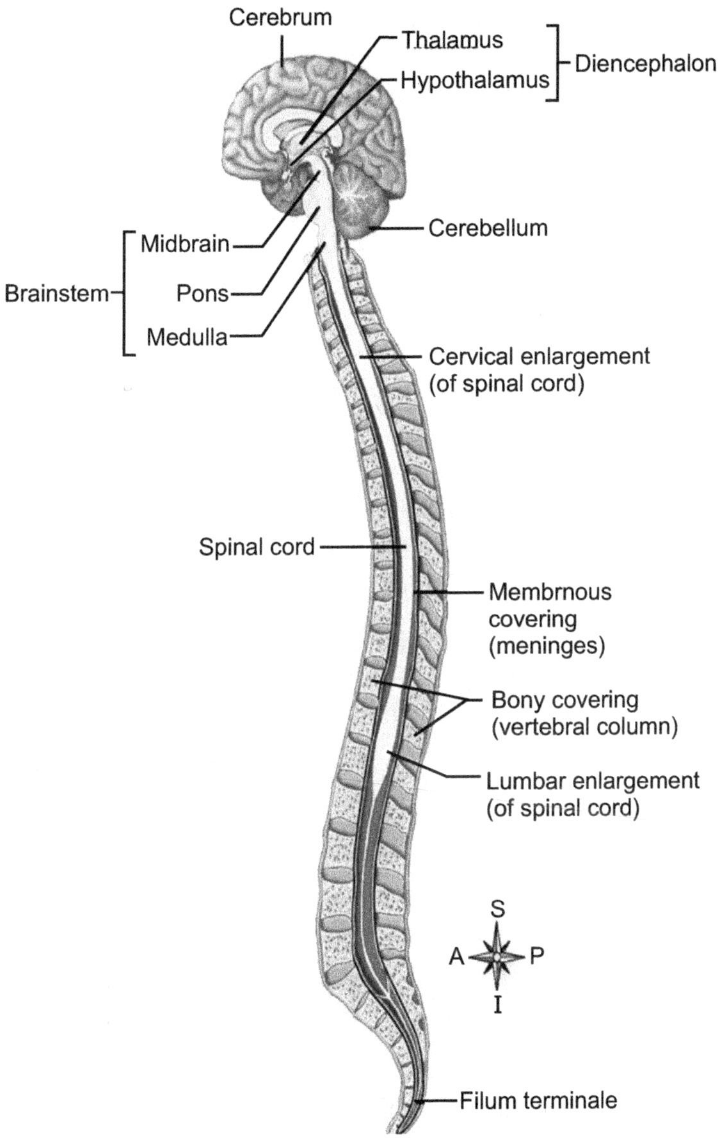

Fig. 3.3: Spinal Cord

Introduction:

A. The central nervous system consisting of the brain and the spinal cord.

B. The peripheral nervous system consisting of:

1. 31 pairs of spinal nerves.
2. 12 pairs of cranial nerves.
3. Autonomic nervous system.

The central nervous system consist of the brain and the spinal cord.

1. Brain consist of:

(i) Cerebrum

(ii) Mid brain

(iii) Pons varoli

(iv) Medulla oblongata

(v) Cerebellum

2. Spinal cord:

It is defined as the nervous tissue link between the brain and peripheral organs of body.

The nervous system detects and responds to changes inside and outside the body. Together with the endocrine system it controls important aspects of body function and maintains homeostasis. Nervous system stimulation provides an immediate response while endocrine activity is, in the main, slower and more prolonged. The nervous system consists of the brain, the spinal cord and peripheral nerves. Organization of nervous tissue within the body enables rapid communication between different parts of the body. Response to changes in the internal environment maintains homeostasis and regulates involuntary functions, e.g. blood pressure and digestive activity. Response to changes in the external environment maintains posture and other voluntary activities.

Cerebrum:

This is the largest part of the brain and it occupies the anterior and middle cranial fossae. It is divided by a deep cleft, the *longitudinal cerebral fissure,* into *right* and *left cerebral hemispheres,* each containing one of the lateral ventricles. Deep within the brain the hemispheres are connected by a mass of white matter (nerve fibres) called the *corpus callosum.* The falx cerebri is formed by the dura mater. It separates the two hemispheres and penetrates to the depth of the corpus callosum. The superficial (peripheral) part of the cerebrum is composed of nerve cell bodies or grey matter, forming the *cerebral cortex,* and the deeper layers consist of nerve fibres or white matter. The cerebral cortex shows many infoldings or furrows of varying depth. The exposed areas of the folds are the *gyri* or *convolutions* and these are separated by *sulci* or *fissures.* These convolutions greatly increase the surface area of the cerebrum. For descriptive purposes each hemisphere of the cerebrum is divided into *lobes* which take the names of the bones of the cranium under which they lie:

1. Frontal
2. Parietal
3. Temporal
4. Occipital.

The boundaries of the lobes are marked by deep sulci. These are the *central, lateral* and *parieto-occipital sulci.*

Functions of the Cerebrum:

There are three main varieties of activity associated with the cerebral cortex:

- Mental activities involved in memory, intelligence, sense of responsibility, thinking, reasoning, moral sense and learning are attributed to the *higher centre.*
- Sensory perception, including the perception of pain, temperature, touch, sight, hearing, taste and smell.
- Initiation and control of skeletal (voluntary) muscle contraction.

Brain stem:

Midbrain:

The midbrain is the area of the brain situated around the cerebral aqueduct between the cerebrum above and the *pons* below. It consists of groups of cell bodies and nerve fibres (tracts) which connect the cerebrum with lower parts of the brain and with the spinal cord. The cell bodies act as relay stations for the ascending and descending nerve fibres.

Pons:

The pons is situated in front of the cerebellum, below the midbrain and above the medulla oblongata. It consists mainly of nerve fibres which form a bridge between the two hemispheres of the cerebellum, and of fibres passing between the higher levels of the brain and the spinal cord. There are groups of cells within the pons which act as relay stations and some of these are associated with the cranial nerves. The anatomical structure of the pons differs from that of the cerebrum in that the cell bodies (grey matter) lie deeply and the nerve fibres are on the surface.

Medulla oblongata:

The medulla oblongata extends from the pons above and is continuous with the spinal cord below. It is about 2.5 cm long and it lies just within the cranium above the foramen magnum. Its anterior and posterior surfaces are marked by central fissures. The outer aspect is composed of *white matter* which passes between the brain and the spinal cord, and *grey matter* lies centrally. Some cells constitute relay stations for sensory nerves passing from the spinal cord to the cerebrum. *The vital centre,* consisting of groups of cells associated with autonomic reflex activity, lie in its deeper structure.

These are the:

- Cardiac centre.
- Respiratory centre.
- Vasomotor centre.
- Reflex centre of vomiting, coughing, sneezing and swallowing.

Cerebellum:

The cerebellum is situated behind the pons and immediately below the posterior portion of the cerebrum occupying the posterior cranial fossa. It is ovoid in shape and has two hemispheres, separated by a narrow median strip called the *vermis.* Grey matter forms the surface of the cerebellum, and the white matter lies deeply.

Spinal cord:

The spinal cord is the elongated, almost cylindrical part of the central nervous system, which is suspended in the vertebral canal surrounded by the meninges and cerebrospinal Fluid. It is continuous above with the medulla oblongata and extends from the *upper border of the atlas* to the lower border of the 1st *lumbar vertebra.* It is approximately 45 cm long in an adult Caucasian male, and is about the thickness of the little finger i.e. below the level of the 2nd lumbar vertebra. This procedure is called *lumbar puncture.*

Result:

Questions

1. Name four principle parts of the brain.
2. Name the sites of cerebro spinal fluid production in the brain.
3. Name the three membranes of brain and spinal cord.
4. Which part of the brain is called as the brain stem?
5. State how many pairs of cranial nerves originate from the brain?
6. Give the three important functions of the hypothalamus.
7. State the three functions of cerebrum.
8. Which part of the brain is the largest part and write a note on lobes of brain?

***

Experiment No. 04

Aim: To study the endocrine system using specimen and models.

Requirements:

1. Model of endocrine system and endocrine glands.
2. Charts of endocrine system and endocrine glands.

Theory:

Human Endocrine System: The human endocrine system modulates several processes of the body by the function of hormones. The endocrine system secretes hormones that control how bodily functions work. Thus, the human endocrine system watches over and coordinates all the systems of the body with the use of hormones.

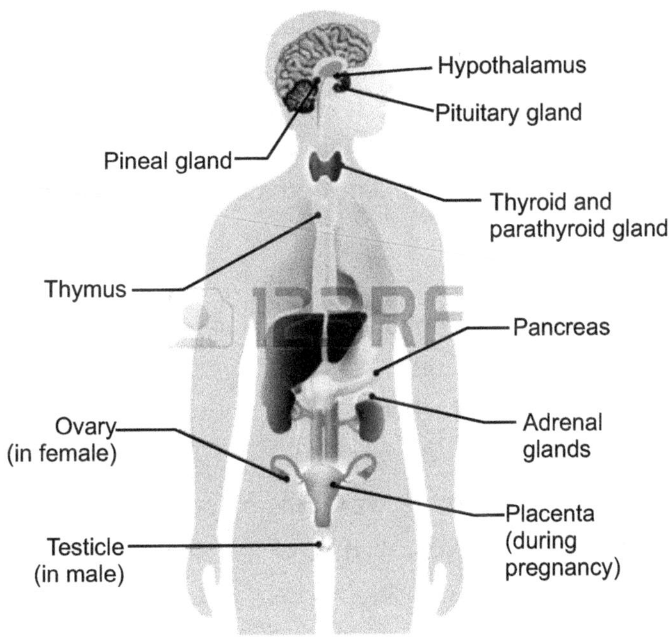

Fig. 4.1: Pituitary gland

Pituitary Gland:

The pituitary gland is located at the base of the human brain. The gland consists of two parts: the anterior lobe (adenohypophysis) and the posterior lobe (neurohypophysis).

The anterior lobe secretes at least seven hormones. One hormone, the human growth hormone (HGH), promotes body growth by accelerating protein synthesis. This hormone is also known as *somatotropin.* A deficiency of the hormone results in dwarfism; an oversecretion results in gigantism.

Another hormone of the anterior pituitary is prolactin, also called lactogenic hormone (LH). This hormone promotes breast development and milk secretion in females.

A third hormone is thyroid-stimulating hormone (TSH). The function of TSH is to control secretions of hormones from the thyroid gland.

A fourth hormone is adrenocorticotropic hormone (ACTH). This hormone controls the secretion of hormones from the adrenal glands.

There are three more hormones produced in the anterior lobe of the pituitary gland. The first is follicle-stimulating hormone (FSH). In females, FSH stimulates the development of a follicle, which contains the egg cell; in males, the hormone stimulates sperm production. The next hormone is luteinizing hormone (LH). In females, LH completes the maturation of the follicle and stimulates the formation of the corpus luteum, which temporarily secretes female hormones. In males, LH is interstitial cell-stimulating hormone (ICSH), which stimulates the production of male hormones in the testes. The final hormone is melanocyte-stimulating hormone (MSH), which stimulates production of the pigment melanin.

The posterior pituitary gland stores and then releases two hormones that are produced in the hypothalamus of the brain. The first hormone is antidiuretic hormone (ADH). This hormone stimulates water reabsorption in the kidneys. It is also called vasopressin. The second hormone is oxytocin, which stimulates contractions in the muscles of the uterus during birth.

Thyroid gland:

The thyroid gland lies against the pharynx at the base of the neck. It consists of two lateral lobes connected by an isthmus. The gland produces thyroxine, a hormone that regulates the rate of metabolism in the body. It also produces a second hormone, calcitonin, which regulates the level of calcium in the blood.

Thyroxine production depends on the availability of iodine. A deficiency of iodine causes thyroid gland enlargement, a condition called goiter. An undersecretion of thyroxine during childhood development results in a condition known as cretinism (dwarfism with abnormal body proportions and possible mental retardation). In adults, an undersecretion can also result in myxedema (physical and mental sluggishness). Thyroxine oversecretion results in a high metabolic rate and Graves' disease.

Parathyroid glands:

The parathyroid glands are located on the posterior surfaces of the thyroid gland. They are tiny masses of glandular tissue that produce parathyroid hormone, also called parathormone. Parathyroid hormone regulates calcium metabolism in the body by increasing calcium reabsorption in the kidneys and by increasing the uptake of calcium from the digestive system.

Endocrine System

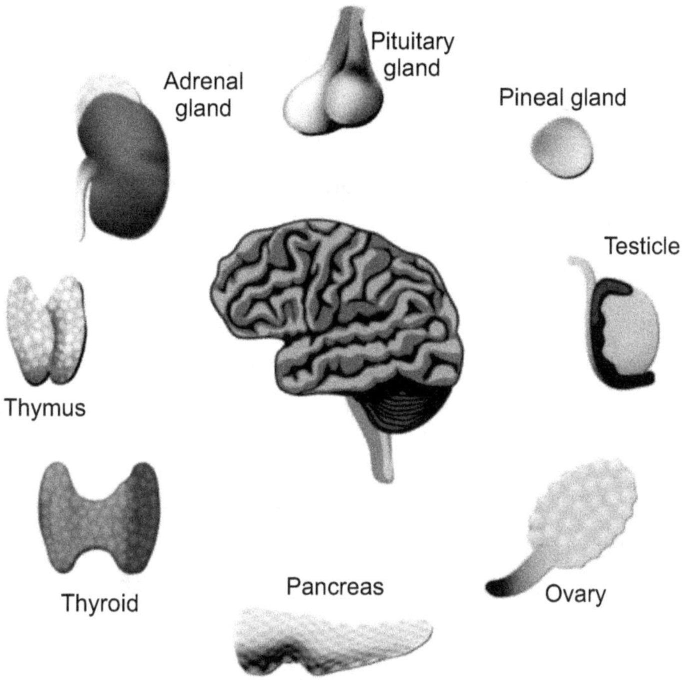

Fig. 4.2: Adrenal glands

Adrenal Glands:

The adrenal glands are two pyramid-shaped glands lying atop the kidneys. The adrenal glands consist of an outer portion, the adrenal cortex, and an inner portion, the medulla.

The adrenal cortex secretes a family of steroids called corticosteroids. The two main types of steroid hormones are mineralocorticoids and glucocorticoids. Mineralocorticoids such as aldosterone control mineral metabolism in the body. They accelerate mineral reabsorption in the kidneys. Mineralocorticoid secretion is regulated by ACTH from the pituitary gland. Glucocorticoids such as cortisol and cortisone control glucose metabolism and protein synthesis in the body. Glucocorticoids are also anti-inflammatory agents.

The adrenal medulla produces two hormones: epinephrine (adrenaline) and norepinephrine (noradrenaline). Epinephrine increases heart rate, blood pressure, and the blood supply to skeletal muscles. Epinephrine functions in stressful situations to promote the fight-or-flight response. Norepinephrine intensifies the effects of epinephrine. Both hormones prolong and intensify the effects of the sympathetic nervous system.

Pancreas:

The pancreas is located just behind the stomach. Its endocrine portion consists of cell clusters called the islets of Langerhans. The pancreas produces two hormones: insulin and glucagon. Insulin is a protein that promotes the passage of glucose molecules into the body cells and regulates glucose metabolism. In the absence of insulin, glucose is removed from the blood and excreted in the kidney, a condition called *diabetes mellitus.* Diabetes mellitus is characterized by glucose in the urine, heavy urination, excessive thirst, and a generally sluggish body metabolism. The second pancreatic hormone, glucagon, stimulates the breakdown of glycogen to glucose in the liver. It also releases fat from the adipose tissue so the fat can be used for the production of carbohydrates.

Other endocrine glands:

Among the other endocrine glands are the ovaries and testes. The ovaries secrete estrogens, which encourage the development of secondary female characteristics. The testes secrete androgens, which promote secondary male characteristics. Testosterone is an important androgen.

The pineal gland is a tiny gland in the midbrain. Its functions are largely unknown, but it seems to regulate mating behaviours and day-night cycles. The thymus gland is located in the neck tissues. It secretes thymosins, which influence the development of the T-lymphocytes of the immune system.

Prostaglandins are hormones secreted by various tissue cells. These hormones produce their effects on smooth muscles, on various glands, and in reproductive physiology. Erythropoietin is a hormone produced by the kidney cells. Erythropoietin functions in the production of red blood cells. Gastrin and secretin are hormones produced by digestive glands to influence digestive processes.

Result:

Questions

1. What is the endocrine system?
2. What is the definition of target tissue?
3. Which hormone stimulates glucocorticoid secretion?
4. Which gland of the endocrine and nervous system controls the other glands in the body?
5. Where is the endocrine system located in the body?
6. What is the endocrine system made up of?
7. How many glands are included in the endocrine system?

***

Experiment No. 05

Aim: To demonstrate the general neurological examination.

Principles:

- Looking for side to side symmetry: one side of the body serves as a control for the other. Determining if there is focal asymmetry.
- Determining whether the process involves the peripheral nervous system (PNS), central nervous system (CNS), or both. Considering if the finding (or findings) can be explained by a single lesion or whether it requires a multifocal process.
- Establishing the lesion's location. If the process involves the CNS, clarifying if it is cortical, subcortical, or multifocal. If subcortical, clarifying whether it is white matter, basal ganglia, brainstem, or spinal cord. If the process involves the PNS then determining whether it localizes to the nerve root, plexus, peripheral nerve, neuromuscular junction, muscle or whether it is multifocal.

A differential diagnosis may then be constructed that takes into account the patient's background (e.g., previous cancer, autoimmune diathesis) and present findings to include the most likely causes. Examinations are aimed at ruling out the most clinically significant causes (even if relatively rare, e.g., brain tumor in a patient with subtle word-finding abnormalities but no increased intracranial pressure) and ruling in the most likely causes.

Introduction:

The goals of the neurological examination are several:

1. **For patients presenting with symptoms suggestive of a neurological problem, the examination should:**
   (a) Determine, on the basis of an organized and thorough examination, whether in fact neurological dysfunction exists.
   (b) Identify which component(s) of the neurological system are affected (e.g. motor, sensory, cranial nerves, or possibly several systems simultaneously).
   (c) If possible, determine the precise location of the problem (e.g. peripheral v central nervous system; region and side of the brain affected etc.).
   (d) On the basis of these findings, generate a list of possible etiologies. Unlikely diagnoses can be excluded and appropriate testing (e.g. brain and spinal cord imaging) then applied in an orderly and logical fashion.
2. **Screening for the presence of discrete abnormalities in patients at risk for the development of neurological disorders:**

This is appropriate for individuals who have no particular subjective symptoms suggestive of a neurological problem, yet have systemic illnesses that might put them at risk for subtle dysfunction. Diabetic patients, for example (particularly those with long standing poor control), may develop peripheral nerve dysfunction. This may only be detected through careful sensory testing (see below under Sensory Testing), which would have important clinical implications.

3. Cursory screening/documentation of baseline function for those who are otherwise healthy:

In patients with neither signs nor risk factors for neurological disease, it's unlikely that the detailed exam would uncover occult problems. Simply observing the patient during the course of the usual H&P (i.e. watching them walk, get up and down from the exam table, etc.) may well suffice. Many examiners incorporate some aspects of the neuro exam into their standard evaluations. Cranial Nerve testing, for example, can be easily blended into the Head and Neck evaluation. Deciding what other aspects to routinely include is based on judgement and experience.

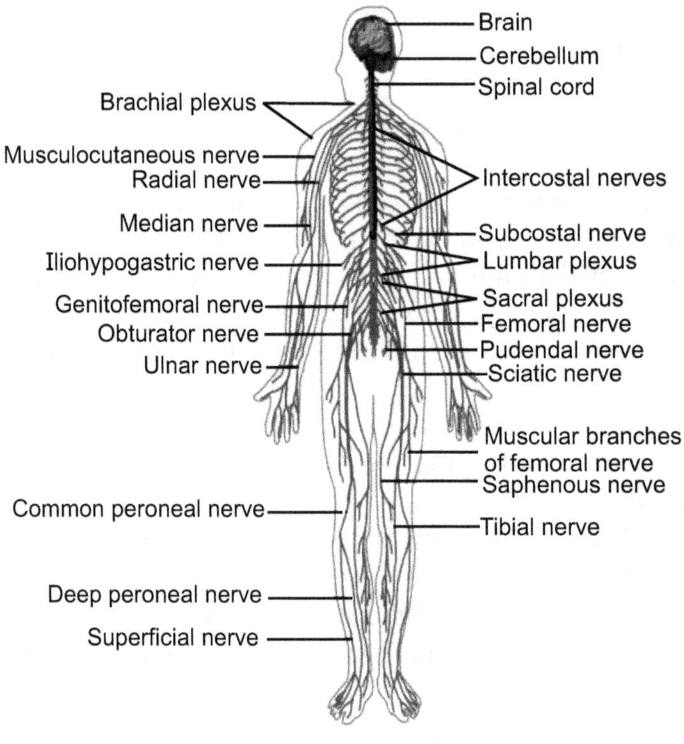

Fig. 5.1: Neurological system

The major areas of the exam, covering the most testable components of the neurological system, include:

1. Mental status testing (covered in a separate section of this website).
2. Cranial Nerves.
3. Muscle strength, tone and bulk.
4. Reflexes.
5. Coordination.
6. Sensory Function.
7. Gait.

Real and imagined problems with the neurological examination:

The neurological examination is one of the least popular and (perhaps) most poorly performed aspects of the complete physical. It is suspected that this situation exists for several reasons:

1. This exam is perceived as being time and labour intensive.
2. Students and house staff never develop an adequate level of confidence in their ability to perform the exam, nor in the accuracy of their findings. This, in turn, probably translates into poor performance later in their careers.
3. Exam findings are often quite subjective. Thus, particularly when the examiner does not have confidence in their abilities, interpretation of the results can be problematic.
4. Understanding/Interpretation of some neurological findings requires an in depth understanding of neuroanatomy and pathophysiology. As many clinicians do not see a large number of patients with neurological disorders, they likely maintain a limited working understanding of this information.
5. There is an over reliance on the utility of neuro-imaging (e.g. CT, MRI). These studies provide an evaluation of anatomy but not function. Thus, while extremely helpful, they must be interpreted within the context of exam findings. Careful examination may make imaging unnecessary. Also, exam findings can make a strong case for the presence of a pathologic process, even if it is not seen on a particular radiological study (i.e. there are limits to what can be seen on even the most high tech imaging).

The above are not meant to lower expectations with regards to how well a physician should be expected to learn and perform the neurological examination. Rather, I mention these points to highlight some of the real and imagined obstacles to clinical performance. Like all other aspects of the physical exam, there is a wealth of information that can be obtained from the neurological examination, provided that it is done carefully and accurately. This is, of course, predicated on learning how to do it correctly.

A few practical considerations/ suggestions:

1. In general, the neurological examination is not applied in its entirety to asymptomatic, otherwise healthy people as the yield (i.e. likelihood of identifying occult disease) would be quite low. It is, however, a good idea to practice the exam early in your careers, even when working with normal patients. This will improve the facility with which you perform the exam, provide you with a better sense of the range of normal, increase the accuracy of the results generated, and give you confidence in the meaning of findings identified when evaluating other patients.
2. It is sometimes appropriate to perform only certain parts of the neurological examination (e.g. just cranial nerves; or only motor testing). These situations will become apparent with experience.

3. The testing described below is still rather basic. There are many additional aspects of the exam that should be applied in specific settings. They are beyond the scope of this text, but can be found in other references.
4. Take advantage of those opportunities when a more experienced clinician examines one of your patients. When possible, watch them perform their exam. Then go back alone and verify the findings.

Like any other aspect of the exam, the neurological assessment has limits. Testing of one system is often predicated on the normal function of other organ systems. If, for example, a patient is visually impaired, they may not be able to perform finger to nose testing, a part of the assessment of cerebellar function (see below). Or, a patient's severe degenerative hip disease will prevent them from walking, making that aspect of the exam impossible to assess. The interpretation of "findings" must therefore take these things into account. Only in this way can you generate an accurate picture. Doing this, of course, takes practice and experience.

Cranial Nerve (CN) Testing:

Many practitioners incorporate cranial nerve testing with their complete examination of the head and neck (see the Head and Neck section of this web site for details). A detailed description of the CN assessment is provided below. As each half of the body has its own cranial nerve, both right and left sides must be checked independently.

Cranial Nerve 1 (Olfactory):

Formal assessment of ability to smell is generally omitted, unless there is a specific complaint. If it is to be tested:

1. Check to make sure that the patient is able to inhale and exhale through the open nostril.
2. Have the patient close their eyes.
3. Present a small test tube filled with something that has a distinct, common odour (e.g. ground coffee) to the open nostrils. The patient should be able to correctly identify the odour at approximately 10 cm.

Cranial Nerve 2 (Optic):

This nerve carries visual impulses from the eye to the optical cortex of the brain by means of the optic tracts. Testing involves 3 phases (also covered in the section of this site dedicated to the Eye Exam):

1. Acuity:

(a) Each eye is tested separately. If the patient uses glasses to view distant objects, they should be permitted to wear them (referred to as best corrected vision).

(b) A Snellen chart is the standard, wall mounted device used for this assessment. Patients are asked to read the letters or numbers on successively lower lines (each with smaller images) until you identify the last line which can be read with 100% accuracy. Each line has a fraction written next to it. 20/20 indicates normal vision. 20/400 means that the patient's vision 20 feet from an object is equivalent to that of a normal person viewing the same object from 400 feet. In other words, the larger the denominator, the worse the vision.

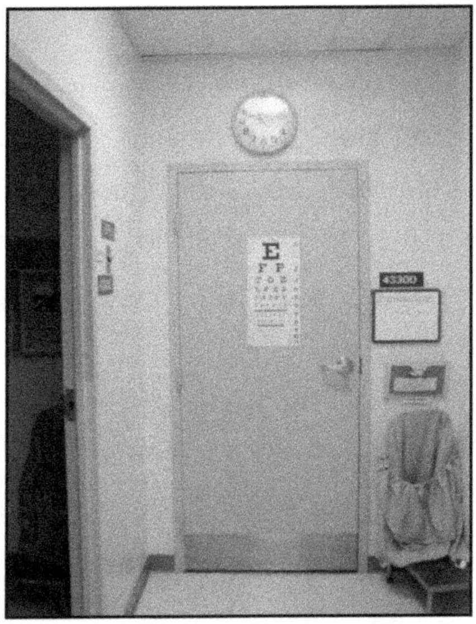

Fig. 5.2: Snellen chart for measuring visual acuity

(c) There are hand held cards that look like Snellen Charts but are positioned 14 inches from the patient. These are used simply for convenience. Testing and interpretation are as described for the Snellen.

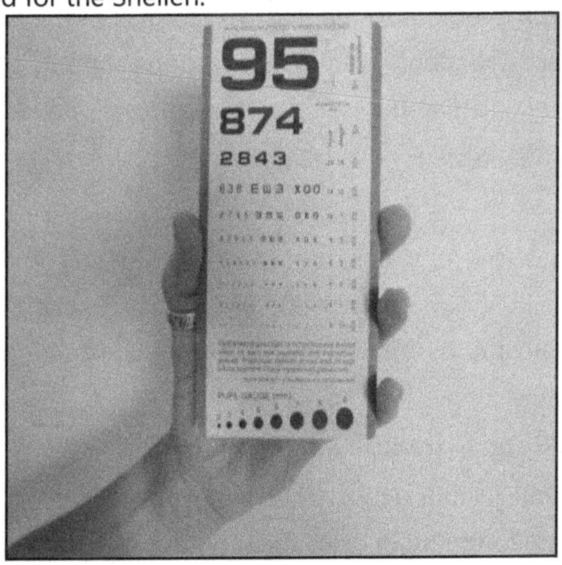

Fig. 5.3: Hand held visual acuity card

(d) If neither chart is available nor the patient has visual complaints, some attempt should be made to objectively measure visual acuity. This is a critically important reference point, particularly when trying to communicate the magnitude of a visual disturbance to a consulting physician. Can the patient read news print? The headline of a newspaper? Distinguish fingers or hand movement in front of their face? Detect light? Failure at each level correlates with a more severe problem.

2. Visual Field Testing:

Specific areas of the retina receive input from precise areas of the visual field. This information is carried to the brain along well defined anatomic pathways. Holes in vision (referred to as visual field cuts) are caused by a disruption along any point in the path from the eyeball to the visual cortex of the brain. Visual fields can be crudely assessed as follows:

(a) The examiner should be nose to nose with the patient, separated by approximately 8 to 12 inches.

(b) Each eye is checked separately. The examiner closes one eye and the patient closes the one opposite. The open eyes should then be staring directly at one another.

(c) The examiner should move their hand out towards the periphery of his/her visual field on the side where the eyes are open. The finger should be equidistant from both persons.

(d) The examiner should then move the wiggling finger in towards them, along an imaginary line drawn between the two persons. The patient and examiner should detect the finger at more or less the same time.

(e) The finger is then moved out to the diagonal corners of the field and moved inwards from each of these directions. Testing is then done starting at a point in front of the closed eyes. The wiggling finger is moved towards the open eyes.

(f) The other eye is then tested.

3. Pupils:

The pupil has afferent (sensory) nerves that travel with CN 2. These nerves carry the impulse generated by the light back towards the brain. They function in concert with efferent (motor) nerves that travel with CN 3 and cause papillary constriction. Seen under CN 3 for specifics of testing.

Cranial nerves 3, 4 and 6 and extra ocular movements:

Normally, the eyes move in concert (i.e. when left eye moves left, right eye moves in same direction to a similar degree). The brain takes the input from each eye and puts it together to form a single image. This coordinated movement depends on 6 extra ocular muscles that insert around the eye balls and allow them to move in all directions. Each muscle is innervated by one of 3 Cranial Nerves (CNs): CNs 3, 4 and 6. Movements are described as: elevation (pupil directed upwards), depression (pupil directed downwards), adbduction (pupil directed laterally), adduction (pupil directed medially), extorsion (top of eye rotating away from the nose), and intorsion (top of eye rotating towards the nose).

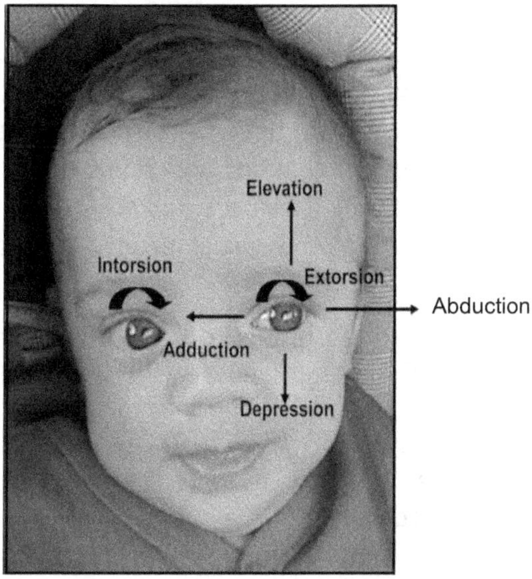

Fig. 5.4: Eye movement terminology

The 3 CNs responsible for eye movement and the muscles that they control are as follows:

- CN 4 (Trochlear): Controls the Superior Oblique muscle.
- CN 6 (Abducens): Controls the Lateral Rectus muscle.
- CN 3 (Oculomotor): Controls the remaining 4 muscles (inferior oblique, inferior rectus, superior rectus, and medial rectus).

EOMs and their function:

The medial and lateral rectus muscles are described first, as their functions are very straight forward:

Lateral rectus: Abduction (i.e. lateral movement along the horizontal plane).

Medial rectus: Adduction (i.e. Medial movement along the horizontal plane).

Table 5.1: Tests in neurological examination

Category	Tests	Example of write up
Mental status examination	• The assessment of consciousness, often using the Glasgow Coma Scale (EMV) • Mental status examination, often including the abbreviated mental test score (AMTS) or mini mental state examination (MMSE) • Global assessment of higher functions • Intracranial pressure is roughly estimated by fundoscopy; this also enables assessment for microvascular disease.	"A & O × 3, short and long-term memory intact"
Cranial nerve examination	Cranial nerves (I-XII): sense of smell (I), visual fields and acuity (II), eye movements (III, IV, VI) and pupils (III, sympathetic and parasympathetic), sensory	"CNII - XII grossly intact"

Category	Tests	Example of write up
	function of face (V), strength of facial (VII) and shoulder girdle muscles (XI), hearing (VII, VIII), taste (VII, IX, X), pharyngeal movement and reflex (IX, X), tongue movements (XII). These are tested by their individual purposes (e.g. the visual acuity can be tested by a Snellen chart).	
Motor system	• Muscle strength, often graded on the MRC scale 0 to 5 (i.e., 0 = Complete Paralysis to 5 = Normal Power). • grades 4−, 4 and 4+ maybe used to indicate movement against slight, moderate and strong resistance respectively. • Muscle tone and signs of rigidity. • Examination of posture • Decerebrate • Decorticate • Hemiparetic • Resting tremors • Abnormal movements • Seizure • Fasciculations • Tone • Spasticity • Pronator drift • Rigidity • Cogwheeling (abnormal tone suggestive of Parkinson's disease) • Gegenhalten – is resistance to passive change, where the strength of antagonist muscles increases with increasing examiner force. More common in dementia.	"Strength 5/5 throughout, tone WNL"
Deep tendon reflexes	Reflexes: masseter, biceps and triceps tendon, knee tendon, ankle jerk and plantar (i.e., Babinski sign). Globally, brisk reflexes suggest an abnormality of the UMN or pyramidal tract, while decreased reflexes suggest abnormality in the anterior horn, LMN, nerve or motor end plate. A reflex hammer is used for this testing.	"2+ symmetric, downgoing plantar reflex"
Sensation	Sensory system testing involves provoking sensations of fine touch, pain and temperature. Fine touch can be evaluated with a monofilament test,	"Intact to sharp and dull throughout"

Category	Tests	Example of write up
	touching various dermatomes with a nylon monofilament to detect any subjective absence of touch perception. • Sensory • Light touch • Pain • Temperature • Vibration • Position sense • Graphesthesia • Stereognosis, and • Two-point discrimination (for discriminative sense) • Extinction • Romberg test – 2 out of the following 3 must be intact to maintain balance: (i) vision (ii) vestibule-cochlear system (iii) epicritic sensation	
Cerebellum	• Cerebellar testing • Dysmetria • Finger-to-nose test • Ankle-over-tibia test • Dysdiadochokinesis • Rapid pronation-supination • Ataxia • Assessment of gait • Nystagmus • Intention tremor • Staccato speech	"Intact finger-to-nose, gaitWNL"

Questions

1. Give principle of neurology.
2. What is the goal of neurological examination?
3. Draw the figure of neurological system.
4. Which problem you face at the time of neurological examination?
5. What is CN Testing?

***

Experiment No. 06

Aim: To demonstrate the function of olfactory nerve.

Requirements:

1. Model of Olfactory nerve
2. Charts of Olfactory nerve

Theory:

The olfactory nerve (Latin: *nervus olfactorius*) is typically considered the first cranial nerve. It contains the afferent nerve fibers of the olfactory receptor neurons, transmitting nerve impulses about odours to the central nervous system, where they are perceived by the sense of smell (olfaction). Derived from the embryonic nasal placode, the olfactory nerve is some what unique among cranial nerves because it is capable of some regeneration if damaged. The olfactory nerve is sensory in nature and originates on the olfactory mucosa in the upper part of the nasal cavity. From the olfactory mucosa, the nerve (actually many small nerve fascicles) travels up through the cribriform plate of the ethmoid bone to reach the surface of the brain. Here the fascicles enter the olfactory bulb and synapse there; from the bulbs (one on each side) the olfactory information is transmitted into the brain via the olfactory tract. The fascicles of the olfactory nerve are not visible on a cadaver brain because they are severed upon removal.

Structure:

The specialized olfactory receptor neurons of the olfactory nerve are located in the olfactory mucosa of the upper parts of the nasal cavity. The olfactory nerves consist of a collection of many sensory nerve fibers that extend from the olfactory epithelium to the olfactory bulb, passing through the many openings of the cribriform plate of the ethmoid bone, a sieve-like structure.

The sense of smell (olfaction) arises from the stimulation of receptors by small molecules inspired in air of varying spatial, chemical, and electrical properties that reach the nasal epithelium in the nasal cavity during inhalation. These stimulants are transduced into electrical activity in the olfactory neurons, which then transmit these impulses to the olfactory bulb and from there to the rest of the central nervous system via the olfactory tract.

The olfactory nerve is the shortest of the twelve cranial nerves and, similar to the optic nerve, does not emanate from the brainstem.

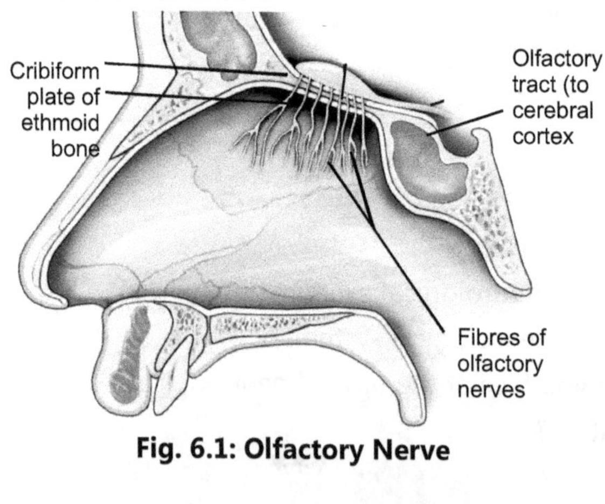

Fig. 6.1: Olfactory Nerve

The functional components of the olfactory nerve include SVA (full form), special visceral afferent, which carries the modality of smell.

Damage to this nerve impairs the sense of smell. To simply test the function of the olfactory nerve, one of the patient's nostrils is closed and a substance with a pungent odour (such as damp coffee essence) is placed under the open nostril. The test is then repeated on the other nostril. If the patient can smell the substance the patient's olfactory nerve is likely functioning. There are olfactory testing packets in which strong odours are embedded into cards and the responses of the patient to each odour can be determined.

Decrease in the ability to smell is a normal consequence of human aging, and usually is more pronounced in men than in women. It is often unrecognized in patients except that they may note a decreased ability to taste (much of taste is actually based on reception of food odour). Some of this decrease results from repeated damage to the olfactory nerve receptors due likely to repeated upper respiratory infections. Patients with Alzheimer's disease almost always have an abnormal sense of smell when tested.

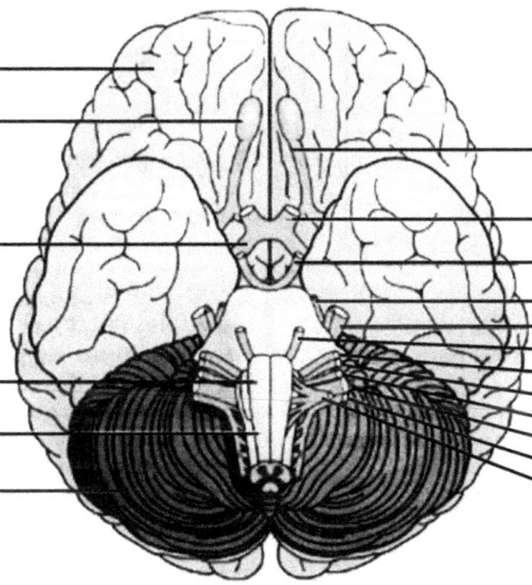

Fig. 6.2: Cranial Nerves

I. Olfactory - Sensory - Smell.

II. Optic - Sensory - Vision.

III. Oculomotor - Motor - Extrinsic eye muscles.

IV. Trochlear - Motor - Extrinsic eye muscles.

V. Trigeminal.

V_1 Opthalmic - Sensory - Cornea, Nasal, Mucosa, Face skin.

V_2 Maxillary - Sensory - Skin of face, Oral cavity, Teeth

V_3 Mandibular - Motor - Muscles of mastication - Sensory - Face skin, Teeth, Tongue (General)

VI. Abducens - Motor - Eye abduction muscles.

VII. Facial - Sensory - Part of tongue (taste) - Motor - Muscles of facial expression

VIII. Vestibulocochlear - Sensory - Hearing, Equilibrium.

IX. Glossopharyngeal - Motor - Stylopharyngeus muscle - Sensory - Tongue (gen and taste), Pharynx

X. Vagus - Motor - Pharynx, Larynx - Sensory - Pharynx, Larynx, abd. organs

XI. Accessory - Motor - Trapezius, Sternocleidomastoid

XII. Hypoglossal - Motor - Tongue muscles.

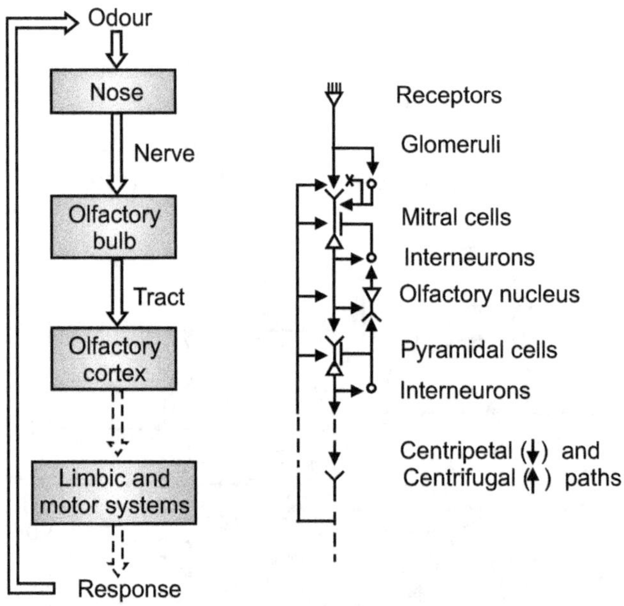

Fig. 6.3: Functioning of Olfactory Nerve

Result:

Questions

1. Where is the olfactory nerve?
2. What are the 12 cranial nerves?
3. What is the olfactory system?
4. Can olfactory nerves regenerate?
5. Which cranial nerves are responsible for blurred vision?
6. What is olfactory dysfunction?
7. Can allergies cause loss of smell and taste?

***

Experiment No. 07

Aim: To examine the different types of taste.

Requirements: Sugar, citric acid, sodium chloride, water, a paper cup, and a tongue depressor or a cotton swab.

Theory:

Taste is the main sensory system that keeps a check on ingested food. Human beings are able to recognize five basic tastes: salty, sour, sweet, bitter and umami. Gustometry (measurement of the acuteness of the sense of taste), including both gustometry with application of taste substances and electrogustometry, is the method of taste examination. There are various methods of applying taste substances during gustometry examination. The stimuli used in gustometry are: citric acid or hydrochloric acid (sour taste), caffeine or quinine hydrochloride (bitter taste), sodium chloride (salty taste), saccharose (sweet taste), monosodium glutamate (umami taste). Electrogustometry, widely used by clinicians to examine taste sensitivity, allows to estimate the functioning of taste by means of electric excitability thresholds determined through the response to the irritation of taste buds area with electrical current of different intensity. Electrogustometry is especially useful in estimating the efficiency of sensory pathways. However, if we want to examine taste sensitivity to individual taste categories we should use more laborious gustometry with the application of taste substances, which main advantage is the use of physiological stimuli.

Taste is the sensation produced when a substance in the mouth reacts chemically with taste receptor cells located on taste buds in the oral cavity, mostly on the tongue. Taste, along with smell (olfaction) and trigeminal nerve stimulation (registering texture, pain, and temperature), determines flavours of food or other substances. Humans have taste receptors on taste buds and other areas including the upper surface of the tongue and the epiglottis.

The tongue is covered with thousands of small bumps called papillae, which are visible to the naked eye. Within each papilla are hundreds of taste buds. The exception to this is the filiform papillae that do not contain taste buds. There are between 2000 and 5000 taste buds that are located on the back and front of the tongue. Others are located on the roof, sides and back of the mouth, and in the throat. Each taste bud contains 50 to 100 taste receptor cells.

The sensation of taste includes five established basic tastes: sweetness, sourness, saltiness, bitterness, and umami. Taste buds are able to differentiate among different tastes through detecting interaction with different molecules or ions. Sweet, umami, and bitter tastes are triggered by the binding of molecules to G protein-coupled receptors on the cell membranes of taste buds. Saltiness and sourness are perceived when alkali metal or hydrogen ions enter taste buds, respectively.

The basic tastes contribute only partially to the sensation and flavour of food in the mouth, other factors include smell, detected by the olfactory epithelium of the nose; texture, detected through a variety of mechanoreceptors, muscle nerves, etc.; temperature, detected by thermo receptors; and "coolness" (such as of menthol) and "hotness" (pungency), through chemesthesis.

As taste senses both harmful and beneficial things, all basic tastes are classified as either aversive or appetitive, depending upon the effect the things they sense have on our bodies. Sweetness helps to identify energy-rich foods, while bitterness serves as a warning sign of poisons.

Among humans, taste perception begins to fade around 50 years of age because of loss of tongue papillae and a general decrease in saliva production. Also, not all mammals share the same taste senses: some rodents can taste starch (which humans cannot), cats cannot taste sweetness, and several other carnivores including hyenas, dolphins, and sea lions, have lost the ability to sense up to four of their ancestral five taste senses.

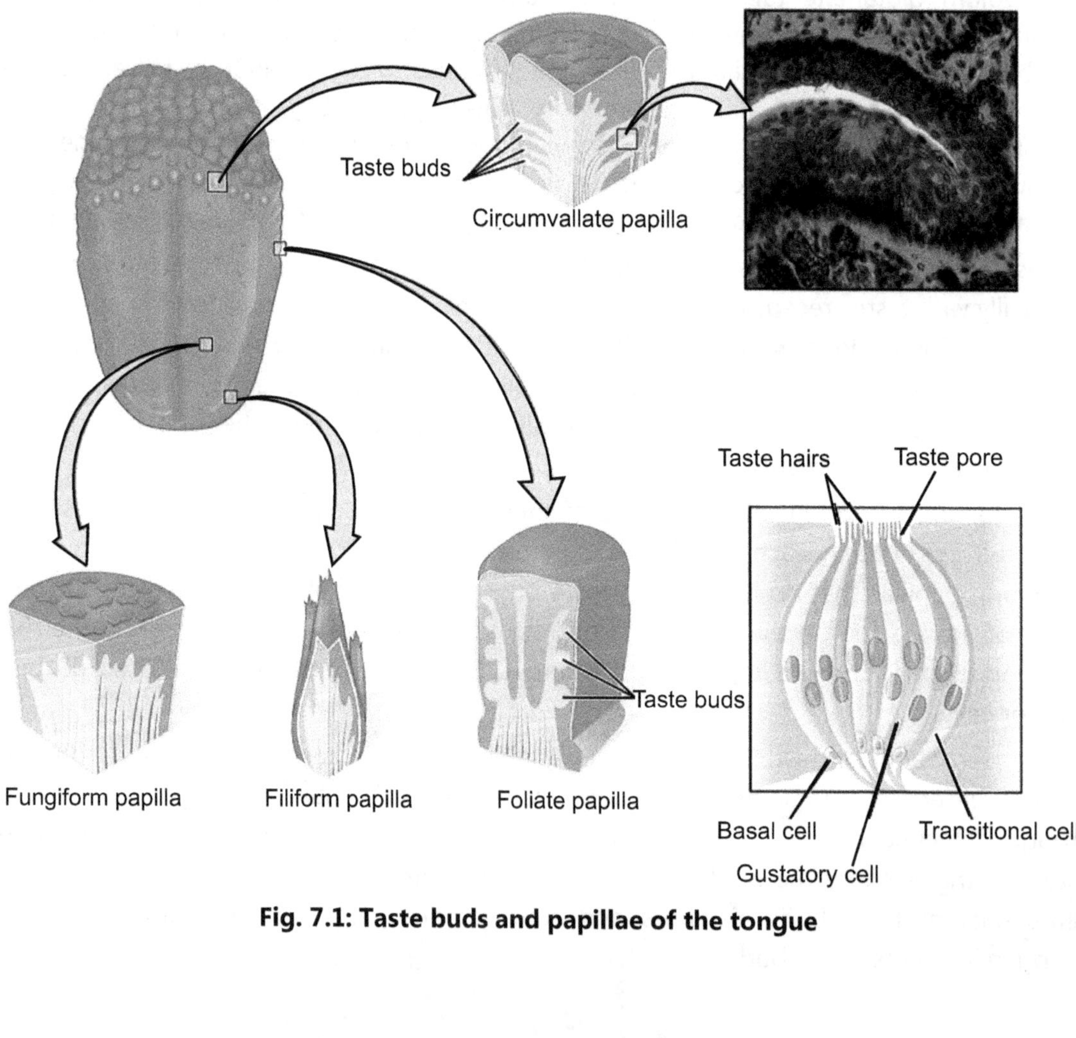

Fig. 7.1: Taste buds and papillae of the tongue

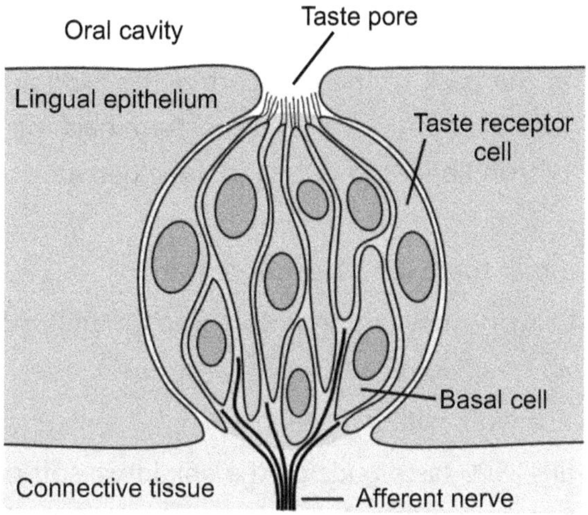

Fig. 7.2: Taste bud

Taste buds and taste papillae:

Taste papillae can be seen on the tongue as little red dots, or raised bumps, particularly at the front of the tongue. These ones are actually called "fungiform" papillae, because they look like little button mushrooms. There are three other kinds of papillae, foliate, circumvallate and the non-gustatory filiform. Taste buds, on the other hand, are collections of cells on these papillae and cannot be seen by the naked eye. To illustrate the point, have a look at the Fig. 6.2. You can see that the taste buds are collections of cells situated on top of, or on the sides of, the different papillae.

In mammals taste buds are located throughout the oral cavity, in the pharynx, the laryngeal epiglottis and at the entrance of the esophagus. Taste buds on the dorsal lingual epithelium are the most numerous (total number of taste buds, all classes, = 4600 per tongue) and best-studied taste end-organs. Here, taste buds are contained within four major classes of papillae.

Types of Papillae:

The majority of taste buds on the tongue sit on raised protrusions of the tongue surface called papillae. There are four types of papillae present in the human tongue:

- **Fungiform papillae:** As the name suggests, these are slightly mushroom-shaped if looked at in longitudinal section. These are present mostly at the apex (tip) of the tongue, as well as at the sides. Innervated by facial nerve.
- **Filiform papillae:** These are thin, long papillae "V"-shaped cones that don't contain taste buds but are the most numerous. These papillae are mechanical and not involved in gustation. They are characterized by increased keratinization.
- **Foliate papillae:** These are ridges and grooves towards the posterior part of the roof of the mouth found on lateral margins. Innervated by facial nerve (anterior papillae) and glossopharyngeal nerve (posterior papillae).

- **Circumvallate papillae:** There are only about 10 to 14 of these papillae on most people, and they are present at the back of the oral part of the tongue. They are arranged in a circular-shaped row just in front of the sulcus terminals of the tongue. They are associated with ducts of Von Ebner's glands, and are innervated by the glossopharyngeal nerve.

  It is generally accepted that there are five taste sensations:

  - Sweet, bitter, and savory (now sometimes called umami), which work with a signal through a G protein-coupled receptor.
  - Salty and sour, which work with ion channels.
  - In addition there are 2500 taste buds on the epiglottis, soft palate, laryngeal and oral pharynx. Many of these taste buds are innervated by the facial nerve (VIIth cranial nerve). The number of taste buds declines with age.

Cells in taste bud:

- **Supporting cells** contain microvilli, appear to secrete substances into lumen of taste bud.
- ***Sensory receptor cell*** has peg-like extensions projecting into lumen. These contain the sites of sensory transduction.
- ***Basal cells:*** These differentiate into new receptor cells. They are derived from surrounding epithelium. The cells are continuously renewed every 10 days or so.

Sweet, sour, salty, bitter and savoury tastes can actually be sensed by all parts of the tongue. Only the sides of the tongue are more sensitive than the middle overall. This is true of all tastes – with one exception: the back of our tongue is very sensitive to bitter tastes. This is apparently to protect us so that we can spit out poisonous or spoiled foods or substances before they enter the throat and are swallowed.

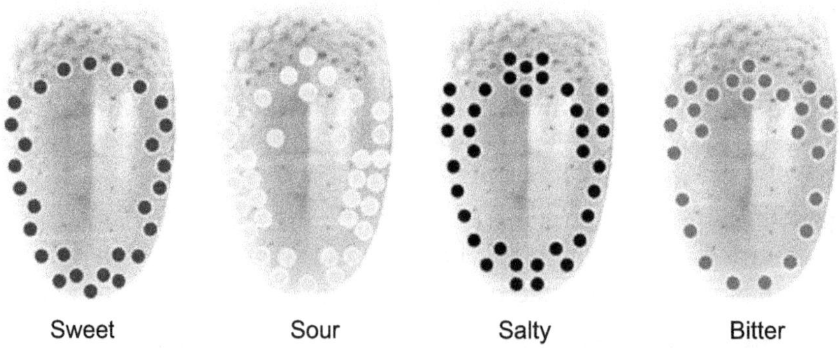

Fig. 7.3: Cells in taste bud

Procedure:

1. Prepare the sugar mixture outside the patients view, so that the contents are unknown. Mix a packet of sugar with a few drops of water so that it has a paste consistency.
2. Explain that you will be testing the patient's ability to taste and that it will not be unpleasant. Ask the patient to close his or her eyes and stick out his or her tongue.
3. Using a tongue depressor or a cotton swab, place some of the paste on one side of the patient's tongue, and ask what he or she tastes.
4. Allow the patient to place the tongue inside the mouth if necessary. Perform the same test on the other side of tongue. If he or she appropriately detects "sweet" or "sugar" on both sides, also ask the patient if the taste is approximately the same on both sides.
5. Repeat the same procedure with other substance to detect taste.

Observation:

Result:

Questions

1. What is the function of taste buds?
2. How many taste buds are on your tongue?
3. Which papillae have no taste buds?
4. Which papillae have the most taste buds?

***

Experiment No. 08

Aim: To demonstrate the visual acuity (VA).

Principal: Optics is the way in which light rays behave as they enter the eye.

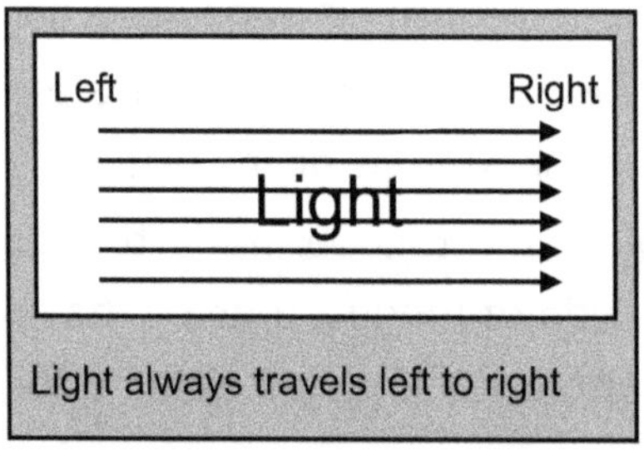

Fig. 8.1: Principal of VA

When light travels, it travels in a straight line. But when light hits the surface of the eye, the lens, some of the light bounces back (reflect) and some of the light will bend (refract).

To understand the principles of refraction, you first need to understand the term "visual acuity".

Visual acuity is how clearly you see an image.

Visual acuity occurs when the light enters the eyes, it is focused directly on to the retina at a single point.

Introduction:

A visual acuity test is an eye exam that checks how well you see the details of a letter or symbol from a specific distance.

Visual acuity refers to the ability to discern the shapes and details of the things you see. It's just one factor in your overall vision. Others include colour vision, peripheral vision, and depth perception.

There are several or different types of visual acuity tests, most of which are very simple. Depending on the type of test and where it's conducted, the exam can be performed by:

1. An optometrist
2. An ophthalmologist
3. An optician
4. A technician
5. A nurse

No risks are associated with visual acuity tests, and you don't need any special preparation.

Definition:

Visual acuity is a measure of the spatial resolution of the visual processing system. VA, as it is sometimes referred to by optical professionals, is tested by requiring the person whose vision is being tested to identify so-called optotypes – stylized letters, Landolt rings, pediatric symbols, symbols for the illiterate, standardized Cyrillic letters in the Golovin–Sivtsev table, or other patterns – on a printed chart (or some other means) from a set viewing distance. Optotypes are represented as black symbols against a white background (i.e. at maximum contrast). The distance between the person's eyes and the testing chart is set so as to approximate "optical infinity" in the way the lens attempts to focus (far acuity), or at a defined reading distance (near acuity).

Purpose of the test:

You may need an eye exam if you feel you're experiencing a vision problem or your vision has changed. A visual acuity test is one part of a comprehensive eye exam.

Children frequently take visual acuity tests. Early testing and detection of vision problems can prevent issues from getting worse.

Optometrists, driver's license bureaus, and many other organizations use this test to check your ability to see.

How the Visual Acuity Test is Performed:

Two commonly used tests are Snellen and Random E.

1. Snellen:

The Snellen test uses a chart of letters or symbols. You've probably seen the chart in a school nurse's office or eye doctor's office. They're different sizes and arranged in rows and columns. Viewed from 14 to 20 feet away, this chart helps determine how well you can see letters and shapes.

During the test, you'll sit or stand a specific distance from the chart and cover one eye. You'll read out loud the letters you see with your uncovered eye. You'll repeat this process with your other eye. Typically, your doctor will ask you to read smaller and smaller letters until you can no longer accurately distinguish letters.

2. Random E:

In the random E test, you'll identify the direction the letter "E" is facing. Looking at the letter on a chart or projection, you'll point in the direction the letter is facing: up, down, left, or right.

These tests tend to be more sophisticated when performed at an eye clinic than in a nurse's office. At an eye doctor's office, the chart might be projected or shown as a mirror reflection. You'll look at the chart through a variety of different lenses. Your doctor will switch out the lenses until you can see the chart clearly. This helps determine your ideal eyeglass or contact lens prescription, if you need vision correction.

Understanding your test results:

Visual acuity is expressed as a fraction, such as 20/20. Having 20/20 vision means that your visual acuity at 20 feet away from an object is normal. If you have 20/40 vision, for example, that means you need to be 20 feet away to see an object that people can normally see from 40 feet away.

If your visual acuity is not 20/20, you may need correction eyeglasses, contact lenses, or surgery. You might also have an eye condition, such as an eye infection or injury, that needs to be treated. You and your doctor will discuss your test results as well as any treatment or correction that might be necessary.

History:

Year	Event
1843	Vision test types are invented in 1843 by the German ophthalmologist Heinrich Kuechler (1811–1873), in Darmstadt, Germany. He argues for need to standardize vision tests and produces three reading charts to avoid memorization.
1854	Eduard Jäger von Jaxtthal, a Vienna oculist, makes improvements to eye chart test types that were developed by Heinrich Kuechler. He published in German, French, English and other languages, a set of reading samples to document functional vision. He uses fonts that were available in the State Printing House in Vienna in 1854 and labels them with the numbers from that printing house catalogue, currently known as Jaeger numbers.
1862	Herman Snellen, a Dutch ophthalmologist, publishes in Utrecht his "Optotypi ad visum determinandum" ("Probebuchstaben zur Bestimmung der Sehschärfe"), the first visual chart based on "Optotypes", advocating the need for standardized vision tests. Snellen's Optotypes are not identical to the test letters used today. They were printed in an 'Egyptian Paragon' font (i.e. using serifs).
1888	Edmund Landolt introduces the broken ring, now known as the Landolt ring, which later becomes an international standard.
1894	Theodour Wertheim in Berlin presents detailed measurements of acuity in peripheral vision.
1978	Hugh Taylor uses these design principles for a "Tumbling E Chart" for illiterates, later used to study the visual acuity of Australian Aborigines.
1982	Rick Ferris et al. of the National Eye Institute chooses the Log MAR chart layout, implemented with Sloan letters, to establish a standardized method of visual acuity measurement for the Early Treatment of Diabetic Retinopathy Study (ETDRS). These charts are used in all subsequent clinical studies, and did much to familiarize the profession with the new layout and progression. Data from the ETDRS were used to select letter combinations that give each line the same average difficulty, without using all letters on each line.

Year	Event
1984	The International Council of Ophthalmology approves a new 'Visual Acuity Measurement Standard', also incorporating the above features.
1988	Antonio Medina and Bradford Howland of the Massachusetts Institute of Technology develop a novel eye testing chart using letters that become invisible with decreasing acuity, rather than blurred as in standard charts. They demonstrated the arbitrary nature of the Snellen fraction and warn about the accuracy of visual acuity determined by using charts of different letter types, calibrated by Snellen's system.

Physiology:

Daylight vision (i.e. photopic vision) is sub served by cone receptor cells which have high spatial density (in the central fovea) and allow high acuity of 6/6 or better. In low light (i.e., scotopic) vision, cones do not have sufficient sensitivity and vision is sub served by rods. Spatial resolution is then much lower. This is due to spatial summation of rods, i.e. a number of rods merge into a bipolar cell, in turn connecting to a ganglion cell, and the resulting unit for resolution is large, and acuity small. Note that there are no rods in the very centre of the visual field, and highest performance in low light is achieved in near peripheral vision.

The maximum angular resolution of the human eye at a distance of 1 km is typically 30 to 60 cm. This gives an angular resolution of between 0.02 and 0.03 degrees, which is roughly 1.2–1.8 arc minutes per line pair, which implies a pixel spacing of 0.6–0.9 arc minutes. 6/6 vision is defined as the ability to resolve two points of light separated by a visual angle of one minute of arc, or about 320–286 pixels per inch for a display on a device held 25 to 30 cm from the eye.

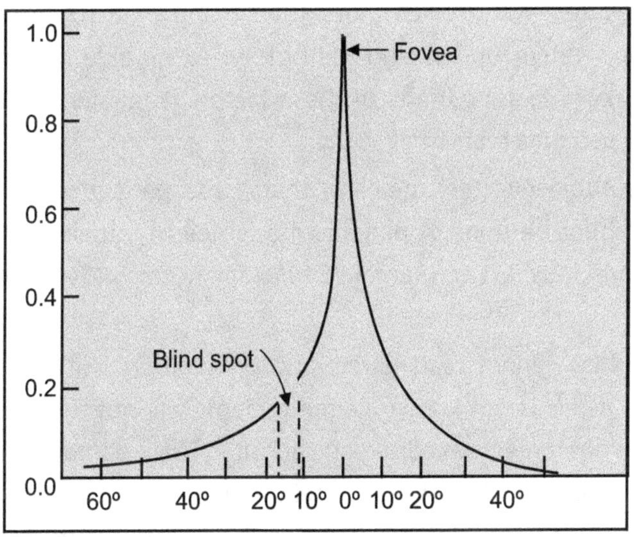

Fig. 8.2: Relative acuity of the human eye on the horizontal meridian in degrees visual angle from foveal vision. The blind spot is at about 18° in the outside direction

Table 8.1: Visual acuity scales

Foot	Metre	Decimal	Log MAR
20/200	6/60	0.10	1.00
20/160	6/48	0.125	0.90
20/125	6/38	0.16	0.80
20/100	6/30	0.20	0.70
20/80	6/24	0.25	0.60
20/63	6/19	0.32	0.50
20/50	6/15	0.40	0.40
20/40	6/12	0.50	0.30
20/32	6/9.5	0.63	0.20
20/25	6/7.5	0.80	0.10
20/20	6/6.0	1.00	0.00
20/16	6/4.8	1.25	−0.10
20/12.5	6/3.8	1.60	−0.20
20/10	6/3.0	2.00	−0.30

Measurement considerations:

Visual acuity measurement involves more than being able to see the optotypes. The patient should be cooperative, understand the optotypes, be able to communicate with the physician, and many more factors. If any of these factors is missing, then the measurement will not represent the patient's real visual acuity.

Visual acuity is a subjective test meaning that if the patient is unwilling or unable to cooperate, the test cannot be done. A patient who is sleepy, intoxicated, or has any disease that can alter their consciousness or mental status, may not achieve their maximum possible acuity.

Illiterate patients who cannot read letters and/or numbers will be registered as having very low visual acuity if this is not known. Some patients will not tell the examiner that they don't know the optotypes, unless asked directly about it. Brain damage can result in a patient not being able to recognize printed letters, or being unable to spell them.

A motor inability can make a person respond incorrectly to the optotype shown and negatively affect the visual acuity measurement.

Variables such as pupil size, background adaptation luminance, duration of presentation, type of optotype used, interaction effects from adjacent visual contours (or "crowding") can all affect visual acuity measurement.

Testing in children:

The newborn's visual acuity is approximately 6/133, developing to 6/6 well after the age of six months in most children, according to a study published in 2009.

The measurement of visual acuity in infants, pre-verbal children and special populations (for instance, handicapped individuals) is not always possible with a letter chart. For these populations, specialised testing is necessary. As a basic examination step, one must check whether visual stimuli can be fixated, centred etc.

Normal visual acuity:

Visual acuity depends upon how accurately light is focused on the retina, the integrity of the eye's neural elements, and the interpretative faculty of the brain. "Normal" visual acuity is frequently considered to be what was defined by Herman Snellen as the ability to recognize an optotype when it subtended 5 minutes of arc, that is Snellen's chart 6/6 meter, 20/20 feet, 1.00 decimal or 0.0 logMAR. In young humans, the average visual acuity of a healthy, emmetropic eye (or ametropic eye with correction) is approximately 6/5 to 6/4, so it is inaccurate to refer to 6/6 visual acuity as "perfect" vision. 6/6 is the visual acuity needed to discriminate two contours separated by 1 arc minute- 1.75 mm at 6 meters.

Questions

1. Define VA.
2. Which test use for VA?
3. Explain history of VA.
4. For children which test is performed.

***

Experiment No. 09

Aim: To demonstrate the reflex activity.

Requirements:

1. Model of Reflex Activity.
2. Charts of Reflex Activity.

Theory:

Definition of Reflex:

Reflex, or reflex action, is the involuntary movement of any organ or body part that has received a stimulus. It happens without any consciousness and is immediate. Reflexes protect the body from harm. For example:

Have you ever burnt got on a stove? What happened when you put your hand on the stove when it was hot? Did you have to say, 'wow that is hot; I need to remove my hand!'? No! You moved your hand immediately because of a reflex.

So how did that reflex happen after you touched the stove? In your hand are nerve endings that pick up a stimulus and carry it to the spinal column and brain. The nerve ending (in this case of burning your hand) is called a sensory neuron (also known as an afferent neuron) because it takes the stimulus - heat to the hand - to the spinal column and brain for interpretation. The brain then interprets the stimulus and sends a message back to the muscles in the hand by a motor neuron (also called an efferent neuron).

The process of the sensory neuron carrying the stimulus to the spinal column and brain, and then the brain sending a message to the motor neuron is called a reflex arc.

Types of Reflexes:

There are several ways to classify the types of reflexes in the body.

First, let's talk about the type or function of reflex. Reflexes can be classified according to the type and function of the muscles or organs that move or function because of the reflex. Some reflexes that move skeletal muscles are called: flexor, extensor, locomotor, and statokinetic. Reflexes that involve functions of internal organs include digestive, cardiovascular, excretory, and secretory.

Next, we can talk about the degree of complexity of the reflex. Reflexes are classified according to the degree of complexity of the neuron (nerve) organization within the reflex arcs.

In this classification, there are monosynaptic (or monosegmental) reflexes, which involve only one segment of the central nervous system, and multisynaptic (or intersegmental) reflexes, which involve more than one segment of the central nervous system.

So let's dive into this topic a bit more. You already know that mono means one and multi means more than one. But, what does that mean in relation to synapses? Monosynaptic means there is only one neuron involved each way on the path to the spinal cord (called an afferent or sensory neuron) and one away from the spinal cord (called an efferent or motor neuron). An example of a monosynaptic reflex is the patellar (knee jerk) reflex.

A multisynaptic reflex, as you can guess, is more complex. In the simplest form, a multisynaptic reflex has more than one neuron (called interneurons) within the reflex arc process. It also involves more than one area of the central nervous system - usually the spinal cord and the brain. An example of this type is the flexor reflex.

Finally, let's look at the influence on muscle or organ of the reflex. Reflexes can have an excitatory (often known as facilitating) action or an inhibitory (weakening and suppressing) activity. For example, we can examine the reflex actions on the heartbeat. The excitatory reflex of the sympathetic nerve will increase the heartbeat. To decrease the heartbeat, or even stop the heartbeat, the vagus nerve is the inhibitory reflex.

Common Reflexes and Examples:

The stretch reflex is one of the simplest reflexes and is monosynaptic. It contracts a muscle that is being stretched and contributes to balance and coordination. A deep tendon reflex is an example of a stretch reflex. How does this work? When you're standing up, your knees bend slightly, and without the deep tendon reflex located around your knees, you could fall. That reflex will straighten your knees and keep you standing upright if you lose your balance. Aside from the knees, deep tendon reflexes are located along the outside of your elbows, in the crooks of your arms, and at your wrists and ankles. This is the same reflex that the doctor checks around your knee.

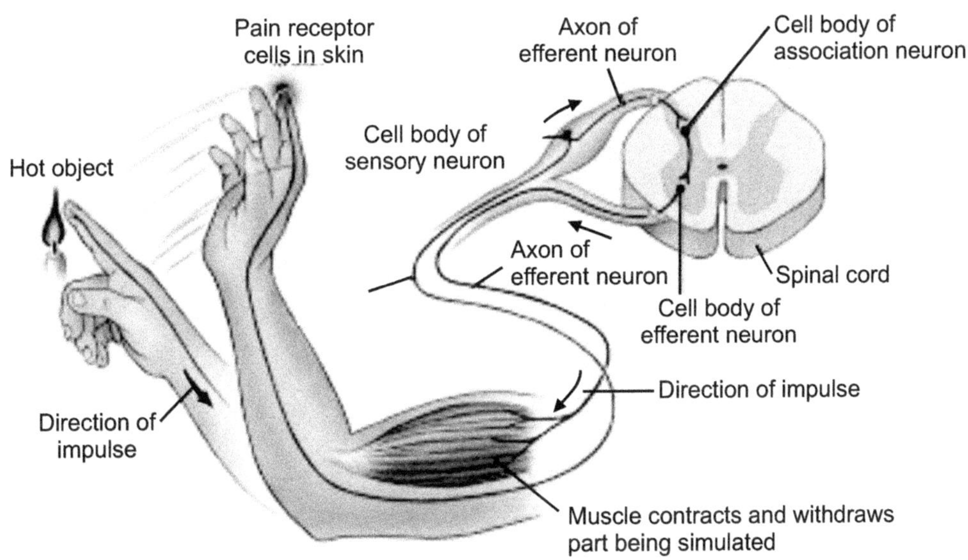

Fig. 9.1: Reflex Action

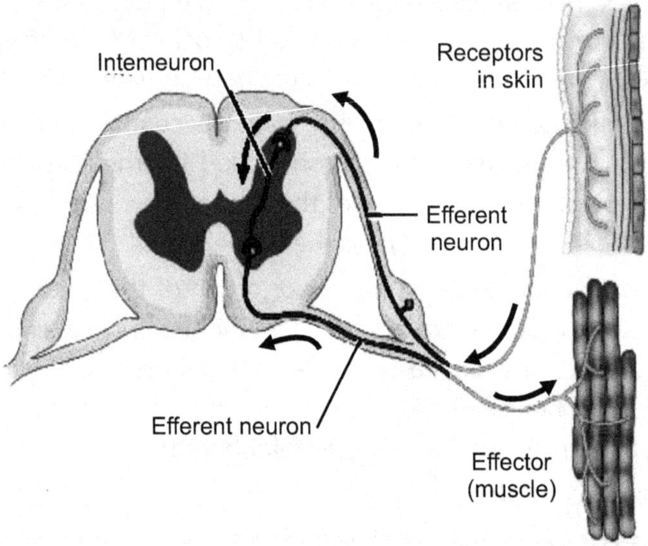

Fig. 9.2: Reflex Action

Result:

Questions

1. Define the term Reflex.
2. Enlist type of Reflexes.
3. Draw the figure of Reflex action.
4. What is the example of Reflexes?

***

Experiment No. 10

Aim: To record the body temperature by using clinical thermometer.

Apparatus:

1. Clinical Thermometer.
2. Stop Watch.

Theory:

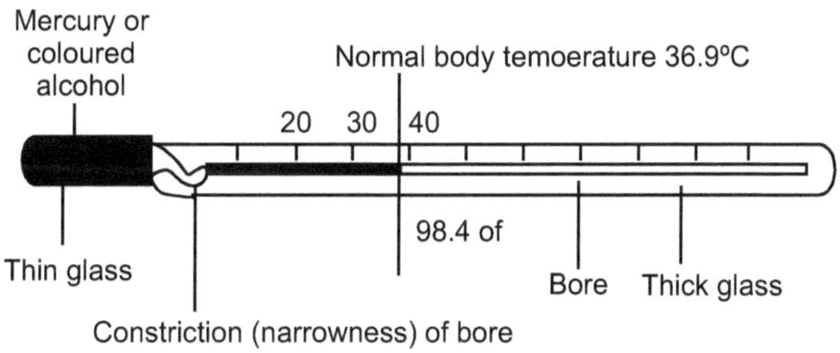

Fig. 10.1: Clinical thermometer

Clinical Thermometer:

Core temperature: The temperature inside the body is called as core temperature. Core temperature is always constant ± 1°F.

Surface temperature: The temperature of the skin tissue underlying the skin is called surface temperature.

Hyperpyrexia: Increase in the body temperature more than normal is called hyperpyrexia.

Hypo pyrexia: Decrease in the body temperature more than normal is called hypo pyrexia.

Procedure:

1. Clean the thermometer with water thoroughly, dip in disinfectant solution for 3 minutes and rinse with water.
2. Dry it with clean napkin.
3. Shake down the thermometer carefully till the mercury below 95°C.
4. Place the mercury bulb in the arm pit or mouth below the tongue.
5. Start the stop watch.
6. Take out the thermometer after half a minute.
7. Read the rise in temperature and record it.

Result:

1. Body temperature is ...... °C.
2. Normal body temperature is 37°C or 97°F.

Conclusion:

1. If the increase in body temperature more than normal i.e. pyrexia or hyperpyrexia.

Significance:

Diagnosis of Hyperpyrexia or Hypopyrexia.

Questions

1. Define fever.
2. Define Hypopyrexia and Hyperpyrexia.
3. State the difference between rectal and oral thermometer.
4. What do you mean by core temperature?
5. Define body temperature.

***

Experiment No. 11

Aim: To demonstrate positive and negative feedback mechanism.

Requirements:

1. Model of feedback mechanism.
2. Charts of feedback mechanism.

Theory:

The biological definition of homeostasis is "the tendency of an organism or cell to regulate its internal environment and maintain equilibrium, usually by a system of feedback controls, so as to stabilize health and functioning". Generally, the body is in homeostasis when its needs are met and its functioning properly.

Every organ in the body contributes to homeostasis. A complex set of chemical, thermal, and neural factors interact in complex ways, both helping and hindering the body while it works to maintain homeostasis.

Homeostatic control: To maintain homeostasis, communication within the body is essential. The image below is an example of how a homeostatic control system works. Here is a brief explanation:

1. **Stimulus** produces a change to a variable (the factor being regulated).
2. **Receptor** detects the change. The receptor monitors the environment and responds to change (stimuli).
3. **Input** information travels along the (afferent) pathway to the control center. The control center determines the appropriate response and course of action.
4. **Output** information sent from the control center travels down the (efferent) pathway to the effectors.
5. **Response:** A response from the effector balances out the original stimulus to maintain homeostasis.

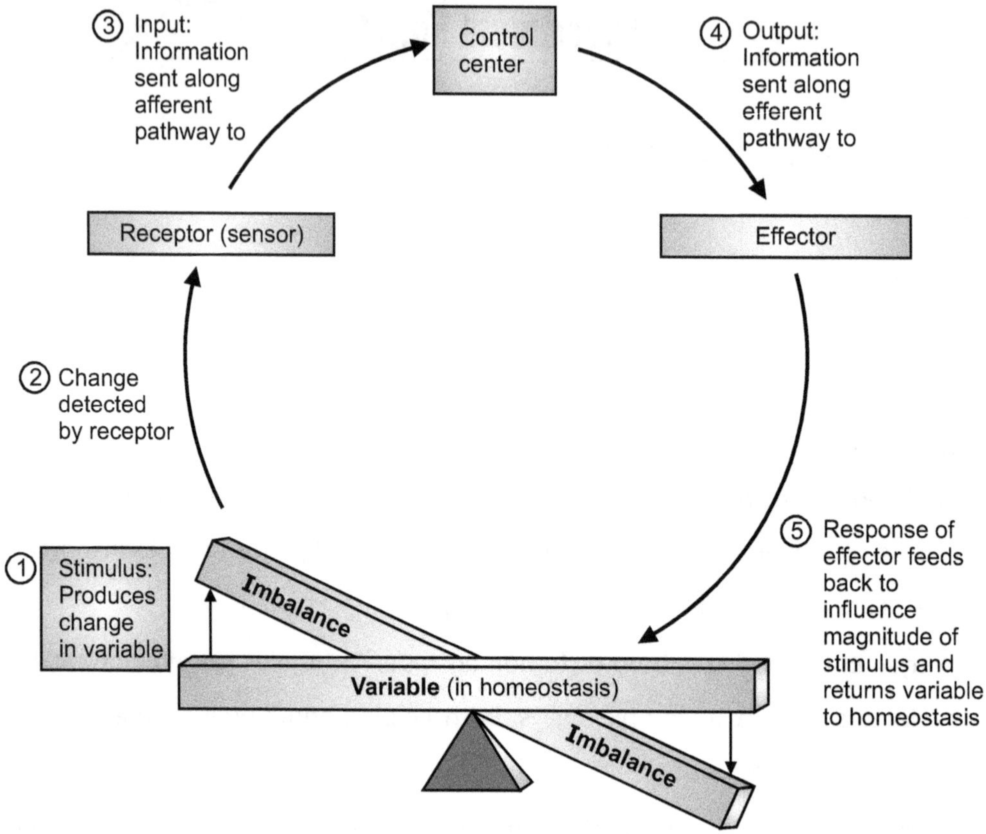

Fig. 11.1: Interactions among the elements of a homeostatic control system maintain stable internal conditions by using positive and negative feedback mechanisms

Think of it as an extremely complex balancing act. Here are a few more definitions you may want to know.

Afferent pathways carry nerve impulses into the central nervous system. For instance, if you felt scorching heat on your hand, the message would travel through afferent pathways to your central nervous system.

Efferent pathways carry nerve impulses away from the central nervous system to effectors (muscles, glands).

The feeling of heat would travel through an afferent pathway to the central nervous system. It would then interact with the effector and travel down the efferent pathway, eventually making the person remove their hand from the scorching heat.

Negative feedback mechanisms:

Almost all homeostatic control mechanisms are negative feedback mechanisms. These mechanisms change the variable back to its original state or "ideal value".

A good example of a negative feedback mechanism is a home thermostat (heating system). The thermostat contains the receptor (thermometer) and control center. If the heating system is set at 70°F, the heat (effector) is turned on if the temperature drops below 70°F. After the heater heats the house to 70°F, it shuts off effectively maintaining the ideal temperature.

The control of blood sugar (glucose) by insulin is another good example of a negative feedback mechanism. When blood sugar rises, receptors in the body sense a change. In turn, the control center (pancreas) secretes insulin into the blood effectively lowering blood sugar levels. Once blood sugar levels reach homeostasis, the pancreas stops releasing insulin.

These are just two examples of negative feedback mechanisms within our body, there are 100's, can you think of a few more?

Positive feedback mechanisms:

A positive feedback mechanism is the exact opposite of a negative feedback mechanism. With negative feedback, the output reduces the original effect of the stimulus. In a positive feedback system, the output enhances the original stimulus. A good example of a positive feedback system is child birth. During labour, a hormone called oxytocin is released that intensifies and speeds up contractions. The increase in contractions causes more oxytocin to be released and the cycle goes on until the baby is born. The birth ends the release of oxytocin and ends the positive feedback mechanism.

Another good example of a positive feedback mechanism is blood clotting. Once a vessel is damaged, platelets start to cling to the injured site and release chemicals that attract more platelets. The platelets continue to pile up and release chemicals until a clot is formed.

Just remember that positive feedback mechanisms enhance the original stimulus and negative feedback mechanisms inhibit it.

Result:

Questions

1. What is a positive feedback mechanism?
2. What are some examples of positive feedback?
3. How does the body use negative feedback to help maintain homeostasis?
4. What is the difference between positive and negative feedback?
5. What are some examples of negative feedback?

***

Experiment No. 12

Aim: Determination of tidal volume and vital capacity by using hutchinson spirometer.

Requirements:

Hutchinson Spirometer

Theory:

While at rest, a healthy adult averages 12 breaths a minute, with each inhalation and exhalation moving about 500 ml of air into and out of the lungs. The volume of one normal breath is called the **tidal volume (VT).** The **minute ventilation (MV)** the total volume of air inhaled and exhaled each minute is respiratory rate multiplied by tidal volume: MV 12 breaths/min 500 ml/breath 6 liters/min.

A lower-than-normal minute ventilation usually is a sign of pulmonary malfunction. The apparatus commonly used to measure the volume of air exchanged during breathing and respiratory rate is a **spirometer** (*spiro-* _ breathe; *meter* _ measuring device) or **respirometer.** The record is called a **spirogram.** Inhalation is recorded as an upward deflection, and exhalation is recorded as a downward deflection. Tidal volume varies considerably from one person to another and in the same person at different times. In a typical adult, about 70% of the tidal volume (350 mL) actually reaches the Measurement of Ventilatory Function Conventionally. A spirometer is a device used to measure time expired and inspired volumes, and from these we can calculate how effectively and how quickly the lungs can be emptied and filled. A spirogram is thus a volume-time curve a typical curve. Alternatively, measures of flow can be made either absolutely (e.g. peak expiratory flow) or as a function of volume, thus generating a flow-volume curve the shape of which is reproducible for any individual but varies considerably between different lung diseases. A poorly performed manoeuvre is usually characterised by poor reproducibility. The measurements which are usually made are as follows:

1. VC (vital capacity) is the maximum volume of air which can be exhaled or inspired during either a maximally forced (FVC) or a slow (VC) manoeuvre. VC is normally equal to FVC unless airflow obstruction is present, in which case VC is usually higher than FVC.
2. FEV 1 (forced expired volume in one second) is the volume expired in the first second of maximal expiration after a maximal inspiration and is a useful measure of how quickly full lungs can be emptied.
3. FEV 1/VC (or FEV1/FVC) is the FEV 1 expressed as a percentage of the VC or FVC (whichever volume is larger) and gives a clinically useful index of airflow limitation.
4. FEF 25-75% is the average expired flow over the middle half of the FVC manoeuvre and is regarded as a more sensitive measure of small airways narrowing than FEV 1. Unfortunately FEF 25-75% has a wide range of normality, is less reproducible than FEV 1, and is difficult to interpret if the VC (or FVC) is reduced or increased.

5. PEF (peak expiratory flow) is the maximal expiratory flow rate achieved and this occurs very early in the forced expiratory manoeuvre.
6. FEF 50% and FEF 75% (forced expiratory flow at 50% or 75% FVC) is the maximal expiratory flow measured at the point where 50% of the FVC has been expired (FEF 50%) and after 75% has been expired (FEF 75%). Both indices have a wide range of normality but are usually reproducible in a given subject provided the FVC is reproducible.
7. FVC 6 is the forced expiratory volume during the first 6 seconds and is a surrogate of the FVC. The FVC 6 (and FEV 1/FVC 6) is gaining popularity because stopping the expiratory manoeuvre after 6 seconds is less demanding and easier to perform for patients with airflow obstruction and the elderly yet is similar to conventional FVC and FEV 1/FVC for diagnosing and grading airflow obstruction. All indices of ventilatory function should be reported at body temperature and pressure saturated with water vapour (BTPS). If this is not done the results will be underestimated, because when the patient blows into a 'cold' spirometer, the volume recorded by the spirometer is less than that displaced by the lungs.

Procedure:

1. Adjust the zero on spirometer.
2. Ask the subject to lay down to measure the vital capacity in supine position.
3. Ask the subject to blow in the pump of spirometer.
4. Record the vital capacity from the scale of spirometer.
5. Ask the subject to sit on the chair and then ask the subject to blow in the spirometer.
6. Record the vital capacity from the scale of spirometer.

Result:

The vital capacity of the subject is found to be ...... in supine position and ...... in sitting position.

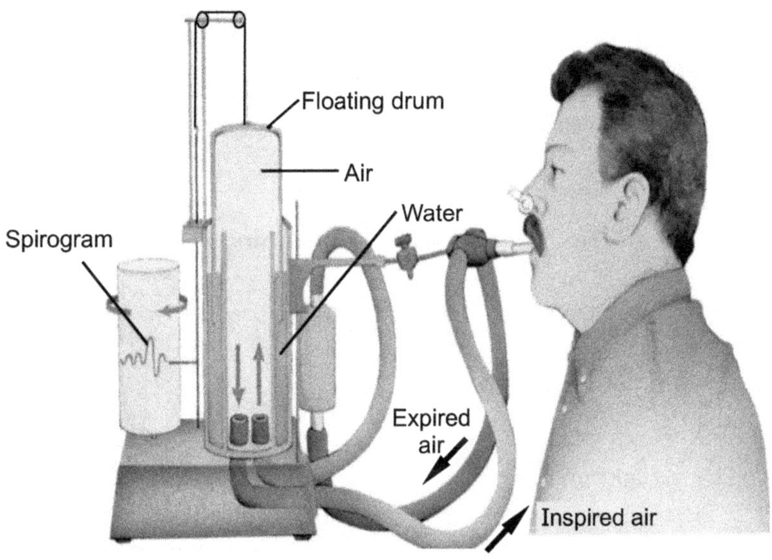

Fig. 12.1: Spirometer

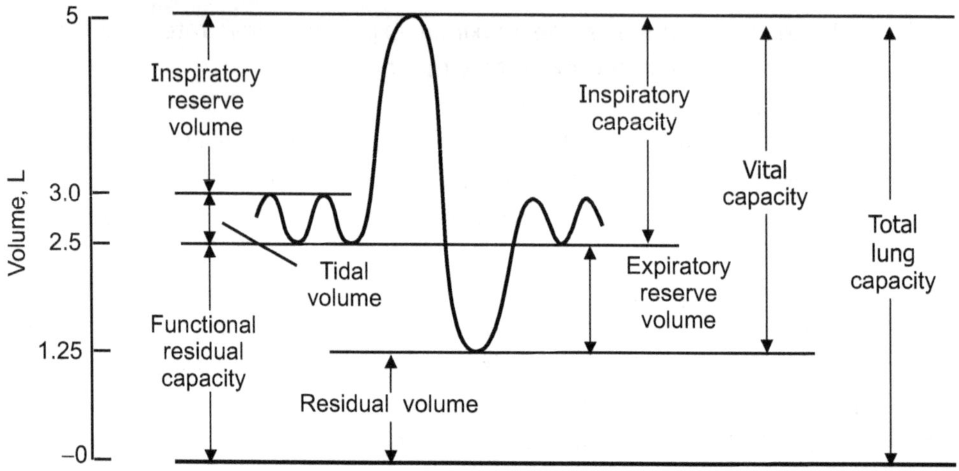

Fig. 12.2: Flowchart of spirometer breathing

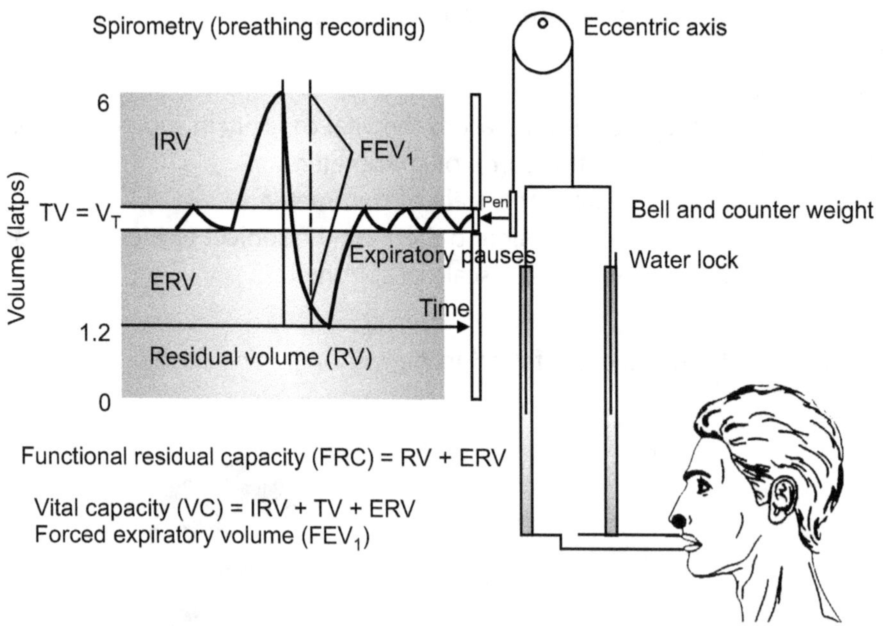

Fig. 12.3: Spirometry breathing

Questions

1. Define minute ventilation (MV).
2. What is spirogram.
3. Draw a well label diagram of spirometer.

***

Experiment No. 13

Aim: To study the structure and functions of digestive system.

Apparatus:

1. Model of digestive system.
2. Chart of digestive system.

Theory:

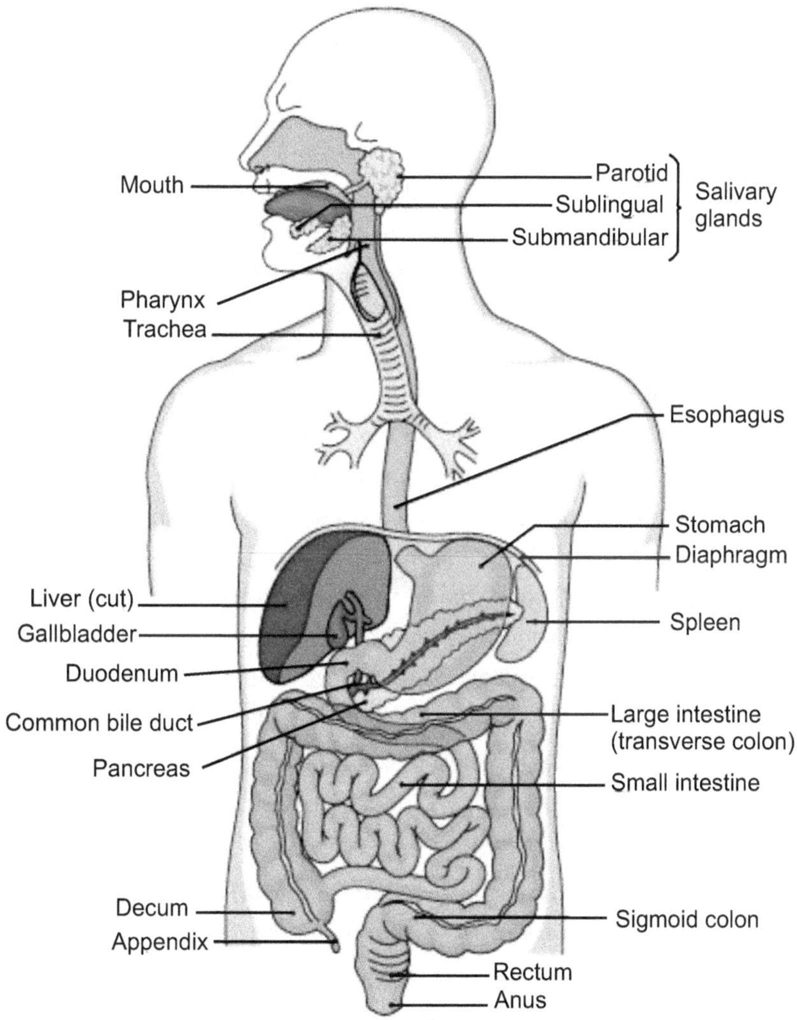

Fig. 13.1: The organs of the digestive system

The human digestive canal is a long tube consisting of following organs:

1. Mouth
2. Pharynx
3. Esophagus
4. Stomach
5. Small intestine
6. Jejunum
7. Large intestine
8. Accessory digestive glands
9. Pancreas
10. Liver

Mouth:

The oral cavity is lined throughout with mucous membrane, consisting of stratified squamous epithelium containing small mucus-secreting glands. The part of the mouth between the gums (alveolar ridges) and the cheeks is the vestibule and the remainder of the cavity is the mouth proper. The mucous membrane lining of the cheeks and the lips is reflected on to the gums or alveolar ridges and is continuous with the skin of the face. The palate forms the roof of the mouth and is divided into the anterior hard palate and the posterior soft palate. The bones forming the hard palate are the maxilla and the palatine bones. The soft palate is muscular, curves downwards from the posterior end of the hard palate and blends with the walls of the pharynx at the sides. The uvula is a curved fold of muscle covered with mucous membrane, hanging down from the middle of the free border of the soft palate. Originating from the upper end of the uvula there are four folds of mucous membrane, two passing downwards at each side to form membranous arches. The posterior folds, one on each side, are the palatopharyngeal arches and the two anterior folds are the palatoglossal arches. On each side, between the arches, is a collection of lymphoid tissue called the palatine tonsil.

Oesophagus:

The oesophagus is about 25 cm long and about 2 cm in diameter and lies in the median plane in the thorax in front of the vertebral column behind the trachea and the heart. It is continuous with the pharynx above and just below the diaphragm it joins the stomach. It passes between muscle fibres of the diaphragm behind the central tendon at the level of the 10th thoracic vertebra. Immediately the oesophagus has passed through the diaphragm it curves upwards before opening into the stomach. This sharp angle is believed to be one of the factors which prevents the regurgitation (backward flow) of gastric contents into the oesophagus. The upper and lower ends of the oesophagus are closed by sphincter muscles.

The upper cricopharyngeal sphincter prevents air passing into the oesophagus during inspiration and the aspiration of oesophageal contents. The cardiac or lower oesophageal sphincter prevents the reflux of acid gastric contents into the oesophagus. There is no thickening of the circular muscle in this area and this sphincter is therefore 'physiological', i.e. this region can act as a sphincter without the presence of the anatomical features. When intraabdominal pressure is raised, e.g. during inspiration and defaecation, the tone of the lower sphincter muscle increases. There is an added pinching effect by the contracting muscle fibres of the diaphragm.

Stomach:

The stomach is continuous with the oesophagus at the cardiac sphincter and with the duodenum at the pyloric sphincter. It has two curvatures. The lesser curvature is short, lies on the posterior surface of the stomach and is the downwards continuation of the posterior wall of the oesophagus. Just before the pyloric sphincter it curves upwards to complete the J shape. Where the oesophagus joins the stomach the anterior region angles acutely upwards, curves downwards forming the greater curvature then slightly upwards towards the pyloric sphincter. The stomach is divided into three regions: the fundus, the body and the antrum. At the distal end of the pyloric antrum is the pyloric sphincter, guarding the opening between the stomach and the duodenum. When the stomach is inactive the pyloric sphincter is relaxed and open and when the stomach contains food the sphincter is closed.

Small intestine:

The small intestine is continuous with the stomach at the pyloric sphincter and leads into the large intestine at the ileocaecal valve. It is a little over 5 metres long and lies in the abdominal cavity surrounded by the large intestine. In the small intestine the chemical digestion of food is completed and most of the absorption of nutrients takes place. The small intestine comprises three main sections continuous with each other.

The duodenum is about 25 cm long and curves around the head of the pancreas. Secretions from the gall bladder and pancreas are released into the duodenum through a common structure, the hepatopancreatic ampulla, and the opening into the duodenum is guarded by the hepatopancreatic sphincter (of Oddi).

The jejunum is the middle section of the small intestine and is about 2 metres long. The ileum, or terminal section, is about 3 metres long and ends at the ileocaecal valve, which controls the flow of material from the ileum to the caecum, the first part of the large intestine, and prevents regurgitation.

The large intestine:

This is about 1.5 metres long, beginning at the caecum in the right iliac fossa and terminating at the rectum and anal canal deep in the pelvis. Its lumen is larger than that of the small intestine. It forms an arch round the coiled-up small intestine. For descriptive purposes the colon is divided into the caecum, ascending colon, transverse colon, descending colon, sigmoid colon, rectum and anal canal.

The caecum:

This is the first part of the colon. It is a dilated region which has a blind end inferiorly and is continuous with the ascending colon superiorly. Just below the junction of the two the ileocaecal valve opens from the ileum. The vermiform appendix is a fine tube, closed at one end, which leads from the caecum. It is usually about 13 cm long and has the same structure as the walls of the colon but contains more lymphoid tissue.

- **The ascending colon:** This passes upwards from the caecum to the level of the liver where it curves acutely to the left at the hepatic flexure to become the transverse colon.
- **The transverse colon:** This is a loop of colon which extends across the abdominal cavity in front of the duodenum and the stomach to the area of the spleen where it forms the splenic flexure and curves acutely downwards to become the descending colon.
- **The descending colon:** This passes down the left side of the abdominal cavity then curves towards the midline. After it enters the true pelvis it is known as the sigmoid colon.
- **The sigmoid colon:** This part describes an S-shaped curve in the pelvis then continues downwards to become the rectum.

The rectum:

This is a slightly dilated section of the colon about 13 cm long. It leads from the sigmoid colon and terminates in the anal canal.

The anal canal:

This is a short passage about 3.8 cm long in the adult and leads from the rectum to the exterior. Two sphincter muscles control the anus; the internal sphincter, consisting of smooth muscle fibres, is under the control of the autonomic nervous system and the external sphincter, formed by skeletal muscle, is under voluntary control.

Pancreas:

The exocrine pancreas

This consists of a large number of lobules made up of small alveoli, the walls of which consist of secretory cells. Each lobule is drained by a tiny duct and these unite eventually to form the pancreatic duct, which extends the whole length of the gland and opens into the duodenum.

Just before entering the duodenum the pancreatic duct joins the common bile duct to form the hepatopancreatic ampulla. The duodenal opening of the ampulla is controlled by the hepatopancreatic sphincter (of Oddi). The function of the exocrine pancreas is to produce pancreatic juice containing enzymes that digest carbohydrates, proteins and fats.

The endocrine pancreas:

Distributed throughout the gland are groups of specialized cells called the pancreatic islets (of Langerhans). The islets have no ducts so the hormones diffuse directly into the blood. The liver is the largest gland in the body, weighing between 1 and 2.3 kg. It is situated in the upper part of the abdominal cavity occupying the greater part of the right hypochondriac region, part of the epigastric region and extending into the left hypochondriac region.

The liver:

The liver is enclosed in a thin inelastic capsule and incompletely covered by a layer of peritoneum. Folds of peritoneum form supporting ligaments attaching the liver to the inferior surface of the diaphragm. It is held in position partly by these ligaments and partly by the pressure of the organs in the abdominal cavity. The liver has four lobes. The two most obvious are the large right lobe and the smaller, wedge-shaped, left lobe. The other two, the caudate and quadrate lobes, are areas on the posterior surface.

Questions

1. State four important functions of Digestive system.
2. Give definition of digestion.
3. Give dental formula for digestion.
4. Give the composition of gastric juice.
5. State three functions of stomach.
6. Give different parts of pancreas.
7. Name four layers of small intestine.
8. Give four functions of liver.
9. Give different parts of large intestine.
10. Name enzymes present in saliva.

***

Experiment No. 14

Aim: To study the structure and functions of cardiovascular system.

Apparatus:

1. Model of human heart
2. Chart of human heart

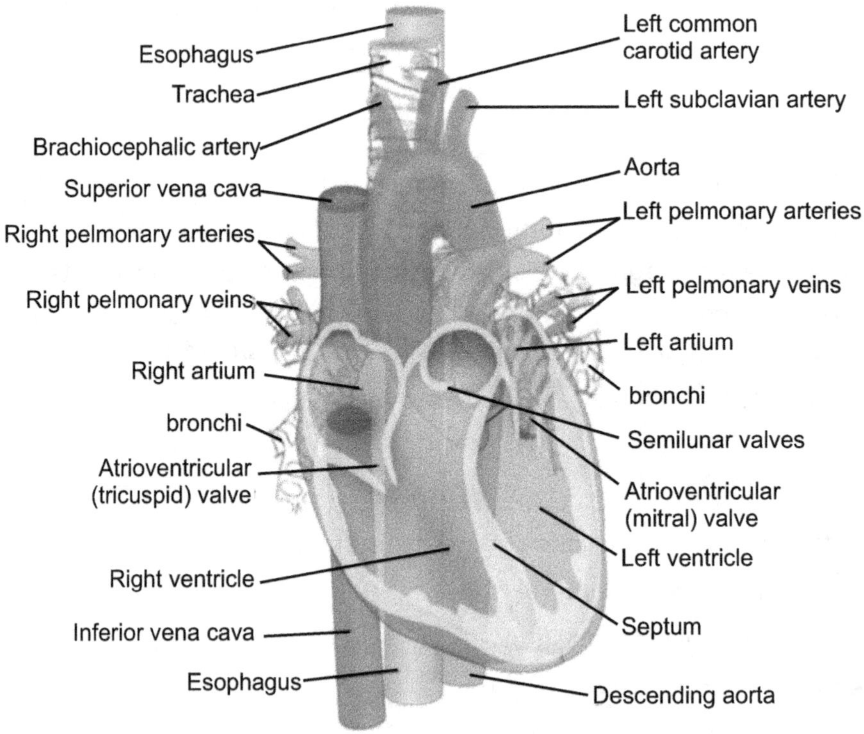

Fig. 14.1: Structure of the heart

Theory:

The human cardiovascular system consist of following parts:

1. Introduction
2. Layers of Heart
   (i) Pericardium
   (ii) Myocardium
   (iii) Endocardium

3. Interior of Heart
4. Conduction system and Sounds of Heart

E.C.G, Cardiac Cycle.

Introduction:

1. Cardiovascular system consist of two main parts of heart and blood vessels.
2. The heart is a roughly cone-shaped hollow muscular organ. It is about 10 cm long and is about the size of the owner's fist. It weighs about 225 g in women and is heavier in men (about 310 g).
3. The heart lies in the thoracic cavity in the mediastinum between the lungs. It lies obliquely, a little more to the left than the right, and presents a *base* above, and an *apex* below. The apex is about 9 cm to the left of the midline at the level of the 5th intercostal space, i.e. a little below the nipple and slightly nearer the midline. The base extends to the level of the 2nd rib.

Layers of Heart:

Pericardium:

The pericardium is made up of two sacs. The outer sac consists of fibrous tissue and the inner of a continuous double layer of serous membrane. The outer fibrous sac is continuous with the tunica adventitia of the great blood vessels above and is adherent to the diaphragm below. Its inelastic, fibrous nature prevents over distension of the heart. The outer layer of the serous membrane, the parietal pericardium, lines the fibrous sac. The inner layer, the visceral pericardium, or epicardium, which is continuous with the parietal pericardium, is adherent to the heart muscle. A similar arrangement of a double membrane forming a closed space is seen also with the pleura, the membrane enclosing the lungs. The serous membrane consists of flattened epithelial cells. It secretes serous fluid into the space between the visceral and parietal layers which allows smooth movement between them when the heart beats. The space between the parietal and visceral pericardium is only a potential space. In health the two layers are in close association, with only the thin film of serous fluid between them.

Myocardium:

The myocardium is composed of specialised cardiac muscle found only in the heart. It is not under voluntary control but, like skeletal muscle, cross-stripes are seen on microscopic examination. Each fibre (cell) has a nucleus and one or more branches. The ends of the cells and their branches are in very close contact with the ends and branches of adjacent cells. Microscopically these 'joints', or intercalated discs, can be seen as thicker, darker lines than the ordinary cross-stripes. This arrangement gives cardiac muscle the appearance of being a sheet of muscle rather than a very large number of individual cells. Because of the end-to-end continuity of the fibres, each one does not need to have a separate nerve supply. When an impulse is initiated it spreads from cell to cell via the branches and intercalated discs over the whole 'sheet' of muscle, causing contraction. The 'sheet' arrangement of the myocardium enables the atria and ventricles to contract in a coordinated and efficient manner. The myocardium is thickest at the apex and thins out towards the base. This reflects the amount of work each chamber contributes to the pumping of blood. It is thickest in the left ventricle. The atria and the ventricles are separated by a ring of fibrous tissue that does not conduct electrical impulses. Consequently, when a wave of electrical activity passes over the atrial muscle, it can only spread to the ventricles through the conducting system which bridges the fibrous ring from atria to ventricles.

Endocardium:

This forms the lining of the myocardium and the heart valves. It is a thin, smooth, glistening membrane which permits smooth flow of blood inside the heart. It consists of flattened epithelial cells, continuous with the endothelium that lines the blood vessels.

Interior of the Heart:

The heart is divided into a right and left side by the septum, a partition consisting of myocardium covered by endocardium. After birth blood cannot cross the septum from one side to the other. Each side is divided by an atrioventricular valve into an upper chamber, the atrium, and a lower chamber, the ventricle. The atrioventricular valves are formed by double folds of endocardium strengthened by a little fibrous tissue. The right atrioventricular valve (tricuspid valve) has three flaps or cusps and the left atrioventricular valve (mitral valve) has two cusps. The valves between the atria and ventricles open and close passively according to changes in pressure in the chambers. They open when the pressure in the atria is greater than that in the ventricles. During ventricular systole (contraction) the pressure in the ventricles rises above that in the atria and the valves snap shut preventing backward flow of blood. The valves are prevented.

Systole:

It is the part of the cardiac cycle when a heart chamber contracts. The term "systole" originates from New Latin, from Ancient Greek (sustolē), from sustellein "to contract" from "together" + stellein, "send".

The mammalian heart has 4 chambers: the left atrium, the left ventricle, the right atrium and the right ventricle.

When the smaller, upper atria chambers contract in late diastole, they send blood down to the larger, lower ventricle chambers. When the lower chambers are filled and the valves to the atria are closed, the ventricles undergo is volumetric contraction (contraction of the ventricles while all valves are closed), marking the first stage of systole. The second phase of systole sends blood from the left ventricle to the aorta and body extremities, and from the right ventricle to the lungs. Thus, the atria and ventricles contract in alternating sequence. The left and right atria feed blood, at the same time, into the ventricles. Then, the left and right ventricles contract simultaneously as well.

Cardiac systole is the contraction of the cardiac muscle in response to an electrochemical stimulus to the heart's cells (cardiomyocytes).

Diastole:

It is the part of the cardiac cycle when the heart refills with blood following systole (contraction). Ventricular diastole is the period during which the ventricles are filling and relaxing, while atrial diastole is the period during which the atria are relaxing.

Cardaic cycle:

It is typically, for a heart rate of 72 beats/minute, a cardiac cycle lasts approximately 0.8 sec, 0.3 sec spent in systole, and 0.5 sec in diastole.

During ventricular diastole, the pressure in the (left and right) ventricles drops from the peak that it reaches in systole. When the pressure in the left ventricle drops to below the pressure in the left atrium, the mitral valve opens, causing accumulated blood from the atrium to flow into the ventricle.

The ventricular filling velocity or flows into the ventricles have two main components; First an early (E) diastolic one caused ventricular suction, and second, a late one created by atrial contraction (A). The E/A ratio can be used as a diagnostic measure, since it is reduced in diastolic dysfunction.

Early diastole, i.e., the E-wave in the E/A ratio, is a suction mechanism. In late diastole, i.e., the A-wave, as the left and right atria contract, the blood pressure in each atrium increases, forcing additional blood into the ventricles. This is known as atrial kick. 80% of the blood flows passively down to the ventricles during the E-wave active suction period, so the atria do not have to contract a great amount.

Stroke volume (SV):

In cardiovascular physiology, stroke volume (SV) is the volume of blood pumped from the left ventricle per beat. Stroke volume is calculated using measurements of ventricle volumes from an echocardiogram and subtracting the volume of the blood in the ventricle at the end of a beat (called end-systolic volume) from the volume of blood just prior to the beat (called end-diastolic volume).

The term stroke volume can apply to each of the two ventricles of the heart, although it usually refers to the left ventricle. The stroke volumes for each ventricle are generally equal, both being approximately 70 ml in a healthy 70-kg man.

Stroke volume is an important determinant of cardiac output, which is the product of stroke volume and heart rate, and is also used to calculate ejection fraction, which is stroke volume divided by end-diastolic volume. Because stroke volume increase in certain conditions and disease states, stroke volume itself correlates with cardiac function.

Cardiac output (CO):

It is a term used in cardiac physiology that describes the volume of blood being pumped by the heart, in particular by the left or right ventricle, per unit time. Cardiac output is the product of the heart rate (HR), which is the number of heart beats per minute, and the stroke volume (SV), which is the volume of blood pumped from the ventricle per beat; thus, CO = HR × SV. Cardiac output values can be represented using many physical units, such as dm^3/min, but is usually denoted as L/min. In a subject weighing 70 kg, the cardiac output at rest would be around 5 L/min; assuming a heart rate of 70 beats/min, the stroke volume would be approximately 70 mL.

Because cardiac output is related to the quantity of blood delivered to various parts of the body, it can be used as an important indicator of how efficiently the heart can meet the body's demands for perfusion. For instance, exercise requires a higher level of CO to support increased muscle activity. In heart failure, CO may be insufficient to even support simple activities of daily living and cannot increase sufficiently to match the higher metabolic demands stemming from even moderate exercise.

Cardiac output is a global blood flow parameter of interest in hæmodynamics, the study of the flow of blood. The factors affecting stroke volume and heart rate also affect cardiac output. The figure to the right illustrates this dependency and lists some of these factors. A detailed hierarchical illustration is provided in a subsequent figure.

There are many methods of measuring CO, both invasively and non-invasively, each with its own advantages and drawbacks. No standard or reference measurement against which all of these methods can be compared exists.

Electrocardiogram (ECG):

An electrocardiogram is a graphic recording of your heart's electrical activity. Simply put, heartbeats are the result of this electrical activity in the cells of the heart. These electrical impulses cause the muscles of the heart to contract and relax in a regular rhythm, creating the pumping action that moves the blood through the body's circulatory system. The ECG records the patterns of that electrical activity. 'Electrocardiogram' is often abbreviated 'cardiogram,' ECG, or EKG (Greek for heart is Kardio, hence the 'K' which is sometimes used instead of a 'C').

Normally, electrical impulses move unimpeded throughout the heart and play an important role in causing the heart to beat. An electrocardiogram can provide considerable information about the health and functioning of your heart. Your doctor can learn about your heart rhythm, the chambers of your heart, the functioning of your heart muscle, whether the heart is enlarged or thickened, and whether you had a heart attack in the past. Abnormalities of the electrical conducting system can also be detected by an ECG.

Questions

1. Give the anatomical position of heart.
2. Name the three layers of heart.
3. Name the valves present in right and left atrioventricular openings.
4. Define cardiac cycle.
5. Define angina pectoris and myocardial infarction.
6. State difference between artery and vein.
7. Give location and properties of cardiac muscle.
8. Define systole and diastole.
9. Define stroke volume.
10. Define cardiac output.

***

Experiment No. 15

Aim: To study the structure and functions of urinary system.

Components of the Urinary System:

Urinary system is one of the most important systems helping maintenance of homeostasis.

The major organs involved in urinary system include:

(A) Two Kidneys : the right and the left

(B) Two Ureters: the right and the left

(C) One Urinary Bladder and

(D) One Urethra

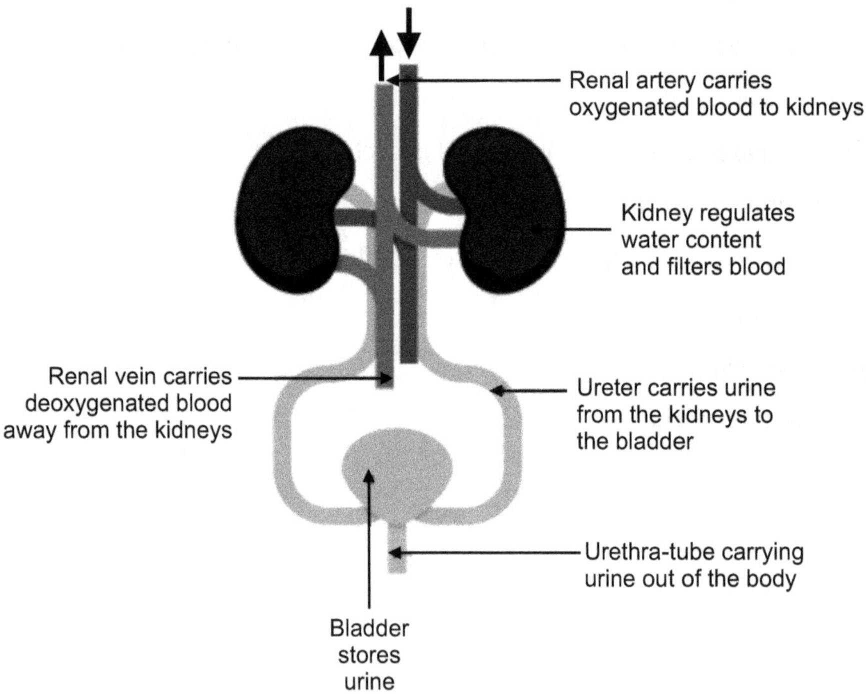

Fig. 15.1: Urinary system

Functions of Urinary System:

In the kidneys, a fluid that resembles plasma is filtered through the glomerular capillaries into the renal tubules (glomerular filtration). As this glomerular filtrate passes down the tubules, its volume is reduced and its composition altered by the processes of tubular reabsorption (removal of water and solutes from the tubular fluid) and tubular secretion (secretion of solutes into the tubular fluid) to form the urine that enters the renal pelvis. From the renal pelvis, the urine passes to the bladder and is expelled to the exterior by the process of urination, or micturition.

1. Regulates blood osmolality, blood volume, blood pressure by altering the volume of water lost in the urine.
2. It regulates the levels of sodium, potassium, chloride, calcium, and other ions by altering the quantity excreted in the urine.
3. By monitoring the hydrogen levels in the blood, this system helps maintain the pH of the body at an optimal level for enzyme function.
4. The kidneys—the major components of this system have endocrine functions. They secrete a hormone (renin) that has an effect on blood pressure.
5. The kidneys also release erythropoietin; a hormone that regulates the production of red blood cells.
6. The kidneys are needed for the formation of vitamin D, an important vitamin required for regulating calcium levels in the blood and proper bone formation.

The Kidneys:

The paired kidneys are bean-shaped with the indentation (the **hilum**) facing medially. The renal artery, renal vein, lymphatics, and renal nerves.

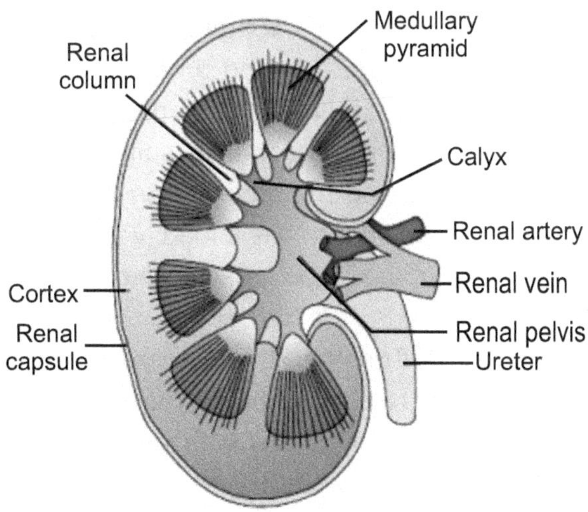

Fig. 15.2: L.S of Kidney

An adult kidney is about 11 cm long, 5–7 cm wide and about 3 cm thick. The kidneys are located on either side of the vertebral column between the T12 and L3 vertebrae. The right kidney is slightly lower than the left because of the presence of the liver. The kidneys are held in place, supported, and protected by the surrounding fat and connective tissue. From deep to superficial, the kidney is invested by a fibrous layer of dense collagen fibers known as the renal capsule. The renal capsule forms a smooth and firm covering to the organ. Medially, the renal capsule folds inward at the hilus and lines an internal cavity, the renal sinus. The renal blood vessels and the ureter pass through the hilus and branch in the renal sinus. The kidney and its vessels are embedded in a mass of adipose tissue (adipose capsule, or perirenal fat). Both the kidneys and the fatty tissue are surrounded by a thick outer layer of fascia, the renal fascia, which anchors the kidneys to surrounding structures such as the peritoneum anteriorly and the fascia covering the backmuscles posteriorly. Because the kidneys are not directly fixed to the abdominal wall, they move with the diaphragm during respiration.

If a section is made through the kidney, it is found to have two distinctive parts:

(i) The outer cortex

(ii) An inner medulla.

Medially, the medulla forms 6–18 conical structures known as renal pyramids. The part of the cortex that dips between the pyramids is the renal column. The apex of the pyramids the renal papilla, located medially projects into the renal sinus. Urine that is formed is drained by the ducts in the papilla into cup-shaped structures known as renal calyx. Four or five smaller calyces the minor calyces empty into two to three larger, major calyces. The major calyces join and form a large chamber, the renal pelvis. The funnel shaped pelvis, which occupies most of the renal sinus, is continuous with the ureter.

The Nephron:

Each kidney is made up of about 1.25 million tubular microscopic structures known as the nephrons. The nephrons are the functional units of the kidney. These nephrons, if laid end to end, would extend about 145 kilometres. Longitudinal Section of the Kidney, Near the Hilum dilated and indented to form a cup. The long tube is the renal tubule, and the cup-shaped end is the glomerular capsule, or Bowman's capsule. Now imagine a network of capillaries nestled in the cup with both ends of the capillaries continuous with a blood vessel—one bringing blood to the cup and the other taking blood from the capillaries. This network of blood vessels is the glomerulus. The blood vessel that brings blood to the capillaries is the afferent arteriole, and the blood vessel taking the blood away is the efferent arteriole. The blood in the afferent arterioles is from the renal artery, which brings blood into the kidney from the abdominal aorta. Together, the glomerular capsule and the glomerulus are known as the renal corpuscle, or malpighian body. The glomerular capsule is a double-walled sac. The outer (parietal) wall is continuous with the inner (visceral) wall where the blood vessels enter. The cavity between the two layers is continuous with the lumen of the tubule. The outer and inner walls are made up of a single layer of epithelium. The visceral layer of the capsule is in close contact with the capillary endothelium and consists of modified epithelial cells (podocytes), with foot like processes known as pedicels. The pedicels wrap around the capillary endothelial cells and the slits between the pedicels (filtration slits) covered by a membrane (slit membrane), permitting the passage of small molecules. The capillary endothelium is leaky, and the endothelial cells contain large pores or fenestrations. These two layers (the visceral layer of the glomerular capsule and the capillary endothelium), together with the basement membrane and the gelatinous, glycoprotein matrix between them, filter those specific substances from the blood that enter the lumen of the tubule. This filter, known as the filtration membrane or the endothelial-capsular membrane. Functionally, the glomerular membrane permits the free passage of neutral substances up to 4 nm in diameter and almost totally excludes those with diameters greater than 8 nm. However, the charges on molecules as well as their diameters affect their passage into Bowman's capsule. Most renal corpuscles are located in the renal cortex. Soon after it forms the glomerular capsule, the tubule becomes coiled—the proximal convoluted tubule. Then it straightens out and descends into the medulla as the descending limb of the loop of Henle, forms a loop (loop of Henle) and goes toward the cortex as the ascending limb. In the cortex, the ascending limb coils again and forms the distal convoluted tubule.

The Renin Angiotensin System:

The kidneys secrete the enzyme renin and renin acts in concert with angiotensin-converting enzyme to form angiotensin II. Angiotensin II acts directly on the adrenal cortex to increase the secretion of aldosterone. Aldosterone increases the retention of sodium from the urine via action on the renal collecting duct. The amount of Na^+ in the extracellular fluid [ECF]) is the most important determinant of ECF volume, and mechanisms that control Na^+ balance are the major mechanisms defending ECF volume. The main mechanism regulating sodium balance is the rennin angiotensin system, a hormone system that regulates blood pressure.

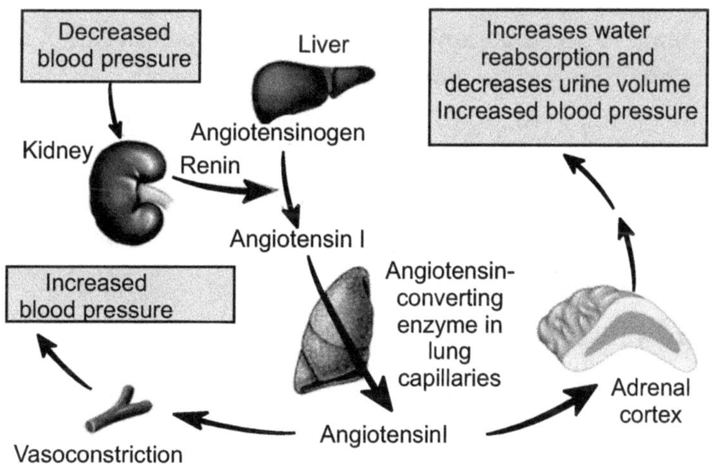

Fig. 15.3: Renin angiotensin system

Renin:

The rise in blood pressure produced by injection of kidney extracts is due to renin, an acid protease secreted by the kidneys into the bloodstream. This enzyme acts in concert with angiotensin-converting enzyme to form angiotensin II.

Angiotensin-converting enzyme (ACE):

It is a dipeptidylcarboxypeptidase that splits off histidyl-leucine from the physiologically inactive angiotensin I, forming the octapeptide angiotensin II. Most of the converting enzyme that forms angiotensin II in the circulation is located in endothelial cells. Much of the conversion occurs as the blood passes through the lungs, but conversion also occurs in many other parts of the body. Angiotensin II is metabolized rapidly; its half-life in the circulation in humans is 1 to 2 min. It is metabolized by various peptidases. An amino peptidase removes the aspartic acid (Asp) residue from the amino terminal of the peptide. The resulting heptapeptide has physiologic activity and is sometimes called angiotensin III. Removal of a second amino terminal residue from angiotensin III produces the hexapeptide sometimes called angiotensin IV, which is also said to have some activity.

Actions of Angiotensins:

Angiotensin I: Appears to function solely as the precursor of angiotensin II and does not have any other established action.

Angiotensin II: Produces arteriolar constriction and a rise in systolic and diastolic blood pressure. It is one of the most potent vasoconstrictors known, being four to eight times as active as norepinephrine on a weight basis in normal individuals. Angiotensin II also acts directly on the adrenal cortex to increase the secretion of aldosterone, and the renin–angiotensin system is a major regulator of aldosterone secretion. Additional actions of angiotensin II include facilitation of the release of norepinephrine by a direct action on postganglionic sympathetic neurons, contraction of mesangial cells with a resultant decrease in glomerular filtration rate and a direct effect on the renal tubules to increase Na^+ reabsorption. Angiotensin II also acts on the brain to decrease the sensitivity of the baroreflex, and this potentiates the pressor effect of angiotensin II. In addition, it acts on the brain to increase water intake and increase the secretion of vasopressin and ACTH.

Angiotensin III: It has about 40% of the pressor activity of angiotensin II, but 100% of the aldosterone stimulating activity.

Juxtaglomerular Apparatus:

The distal convoluted tubule, as mentioned, is in close proximity to its own glomerulus before it straightens and connects with the collecting duct. In this region, the wall of the afferent arteriole, the cells lining the tubule and other cells in the vicinity are modified to form the juxtaglomerular apparatus.

The juxtaglomerular apparatus is an endocrine structure that secretes the erythropoietin and renin. Erythropoietin is a hormone that regulates the production of red blood cells by the bone marrow. The hormone renin is involved with the regulation of blood pressure. The rate of secretion of these hormones is related to the composition of blood in the afferent arteriole and the tubular fluid in the distal convoluted tubule. In this way, if the oxygen content of blood is low, cell production is stimulated by erythropoietin. Similarly, if the blood pressure drops in the renal vessels, it is brought to normal by the actions of renin.

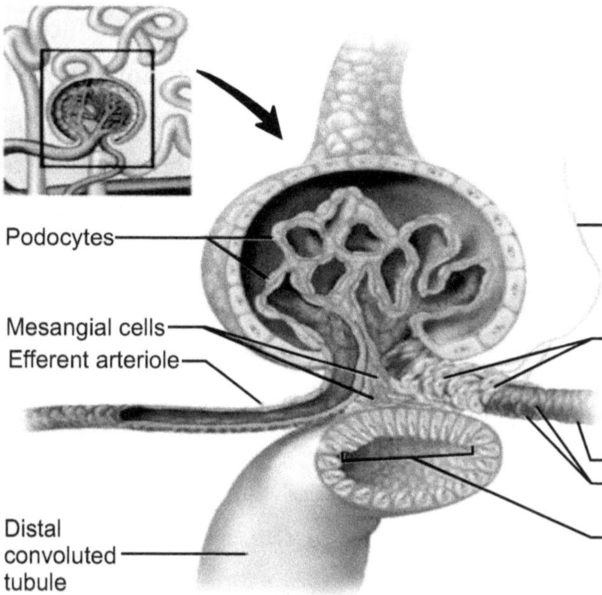

Fig. 15.4: Juxtaglomerular apparatus

Juxtamedullary nephrons:

Although 85% of the nephrons are located in the cortex, 15% of the nephrons are located in the junction of the cortex and the medulla. These nephrons, the juxtamedullary nephrons, have long loops of Henle that descend deep into the medulla. These nephrons, together with the surrounding bloodvessels, play an important role in concentrating urine and conserving water.

Blood Supply to the Kidneys: The right and left renal arteries, branches of the abdominal aorta, supply the kidneys. They bring about 20% to 25% of the total cardiac output (appox., 1.2 Liter per min).

Nerve Supply to the Kidneys: The renal nerves of the sympathetic nervous system are the major nerves that supply the kidneys. These nerves regulate the blood flow and pressure in the glomerulus by controlling the diameter of the afferent and efferent arterioles. They also stimulate the release of renin from the juxtaglomerular apparatus when the blood pressure drops in the body.

Hormones Affecting Kidney Function:

Two hormones play a major part in altering urine concentration. The antidiuretic hormone (ADH), also known as vasopressin, from the posterior pituitary has an effect on the collecting tubules, increasing the reabsorption of water back into the capillaries. The secretion of ADH is increased when the volume of blood decreases. By reducing the volume of water lost in the urine, the body tries to bring about homeostasis. Antidiuretic hormone, in addition, stimulates the thirst center in the brain to increase water intake and constricts blood vessels to increase blood pressure. Aldosterone, another hormone secreted by the adrenal cortex, plays an important role in kidney function. This hormone regulates the sodium content in the blood by altering the amount of sodium reabsorbed by the kidney tubules. In conjunction with ADH, by increasing sodium absorption, it draws water back into the renal capillaries by osmosis.

Physiology of Urine Formation:

The steps in Urine Formation are:

1. Glomerular Filtration.
2. Tubular Reabsorption and
3. Tubular secretion.

1. Glomerular Filtration:

The blood forcefully enters the capillaries of the glomerulus. This blood pressure forces the dissolved blood components and water through the endothelial pores, basement membrane and the slit membranes between the pedicels. Passing through all these layers the fluid expels into the capsular space. This fluid is called glomerular filtrate. In the renal corpuscle, substances from the blood are allowed to pass passively through the filtration membrane, based on their size. Therefore, solutes, such as glucose, amino acids, and fatty acids, are also filtered. Net Filtration Pressure depends upon three different pressures.

- **(a) Glomerular blood hydrostatic pressure:** It is the pressure exerted by blood on the walls of capillaries. It is about 55 mm Hg. This pressure favours the filtration.
- **(b) Capsular hydrostatic pressure:** The fluid as enters the capsular space, it is opposed by the walls of the capsule as well as the fluid already present in the capsular space. And because of this the same fluid is forced back in to the capillaries. It is about 15 mm Hg. This pressure opposes the filtration.
- **(c) Colloidal osmotic pressure of blood:** The plasma proteins and the formed component of the blood exert this opposing pressure. It is about 30 mm Hg. This pressure opposes the filtration.

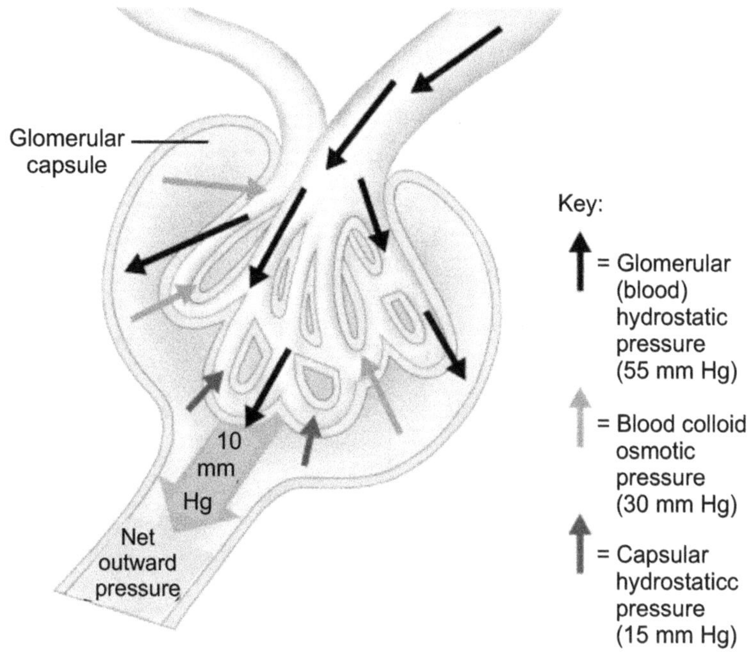

Fig. 15.5: Glomerular Filtration

Hence, the Net Filtration Pressure is = (55 mm Hg) – (15 mm Hg + 30 mm Hg) = 10 mm Hg

The rate at which the glomeruli filter the plasma is called as glomerular filtration rate (GFR) which is 125 mL/minute. The rate of water and electrolyte absorption is modified by the action of hormones such as antidiuretic hormone (ADH) and aldosterone.

2. Tubular Reabsorption:

The filtrate originally formed in the renal corpuscle undergoes many changes as it travels down the renal tubule, according to the internal environment (i.e., in accordance to the blood volume, blood pressure, plasma concentration, and level of such electrolytes as sodium, potassium, and calcium). As this glomerular filtrate passes down the tubules, its volume is reduced and its composition altered by the processes of tubular reabsorption (reabsorption of water and useful solutes).

Water is reabsorbed by osmosis. This drastically reduces the volume of the filtrate. As the fluid descends further into the descending limb, more water is reabsorbed and the tubular fluid becomes concentrated. In the proximal convoluted tubule, most ions and organic substances are actively or passively reabsorbed. Some reabsorbed solutes include sodium, potassium, calcium, chloride, phosphate, and bicarbonate. Small proteins and peptides are reabsorbed by pinocytosis. About 99% of the glomerular filtrate is reabsorbed and only 1% is excreted as urine.

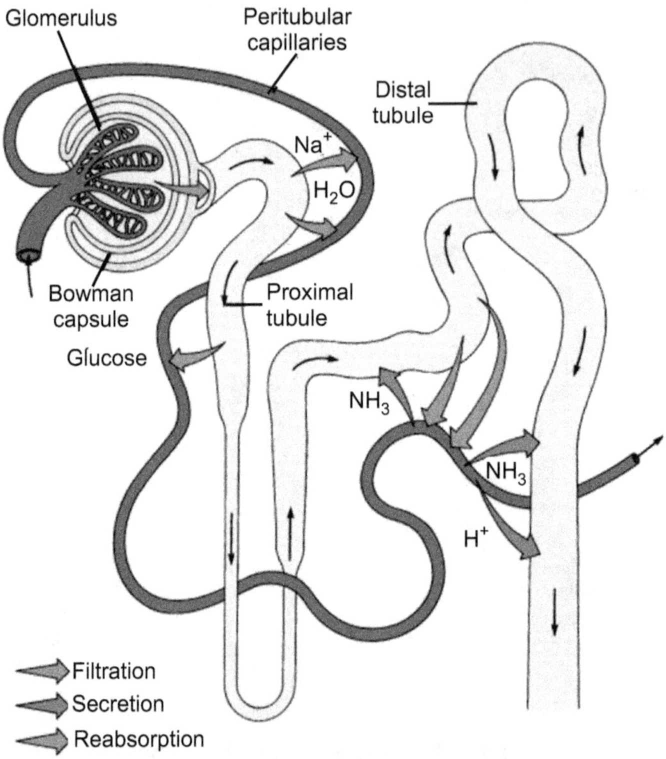

Fig. 15.6: Tubular reabsorption

It emphasizes the manner by which water and important electrolytes and metabolites are conserved. Furthermore, the composition of the urine can be varied to maintain whole body fluid homeostasis (extracellular fluid [ECF]). This is achieved via many homeostatic regulatory mechanisms that function to change the amount of water and solutes in the urine.

3. Tubular secretion:

Secretion of solutes into the tubular fluid to form the urine that enters the renal pelvis. Few substances, such as hydrogen ions, urea, ammonia, and creatinine, may be secreted.

The kidney is important in acid-base balance (pH balance). It can regulate the body pH by conserving or eliminating the bases (e.g., bicarbonate) or acids (e.g., hydrogen ions). The kidney has the capacity to secrete hydrogen ions into the tubular fluid. The three major urinary buffers are:

(i) Bicarbonate (HCO_3):

Bicarbonate present in the filtrate combines with hydrogen ions to form carbonic acid (a weak acid). This acid dissociates into water and carbon dioxide. The carbon dioxide diffuses into the cells and is used to form more bicarbonate ions

$$H^+ \quad + \quad HCO_3^- \longrightarrow H_2CO_3 \rightarrow H_2O + CO_2$$

Hydrogen ion + Bicarbonate ion ⟶ Carbonic Acid ⟶ Water + Carbon dioxide

(ii) Phosphate (HPO_4):

Similarly, filtered phosphate combines with the secreted hydrogen ions and is excreted.

$$H^+ \quad + \quad HPO_3^{2-} \longrightarrow H_2PO_3^-$$

Hydrogen ion + Hydrogen Phosphate ion ⟶ Dihydrogen Phosphate

(iii) Ammonia (NH_3):

The tubular cells manufacture ammonia from the amino acid glutamine. The ammonia combines with hydrogen ions and is also excreted. When the blood pH is alkaline, fewer hydrogen ions are secreted and more bases excreted.

$$H^+ + NH_3 \longrightarrow NH_4^+$$

Hydrogen ion + Ammonia ⟶ Ammonium Ions

In summary, three physical processes simple filtration, selective absorption, and secretion

Composition of Urine:

1. Urine is composed of 93% to 97% water. Urine pH ranges from 4.5–8.0. Normally, about 1,200 mL of urine is excreted each day.
2. Some organic substances present include urea, creatinine, ammonia, uric acid, urobilin, and bilirubin.

(i) Urea is derived from the metabolism of amino acids by the liver and kidneys.

(ii) Creatinine:

It is derived from the breakdown of creatine phosphate in skeletal muscle. Its excretion is proportional to the skeletal muscle mass.

(iii) Ammonia:

It is derived largely from protein breakdown.

(iv) Uric acid:

It is derived from breakdown of nucleic acid, present in large amounts in the nucleus of cells.

(v) Urobilin and bilirubin:

These are breakdown products of hemoglobin and give urine its yellow colour. Increased amounts are excreted when there is liver disease or when there is excessive breakdown of red blood cells.

3. The excretion of sodium, chloride, potassium, sulphate, magnesium, calcium and other ions vary with diet, pH of urine, and effect of hormones.

Ureter and Urinary Bladder:

The function of the bladder is to temporarily store urine which comes from ureter. It is a hollow muscular organ, which is held in place by connective tissue that attaches it to the walls of the pelvic cavity.

Urethra:

The urethra extends from the neck of the bladder to the external urethral opening, or external urethral meatus.

Important Points:

(a) Plasma enters the kidneys and is filtered in the glomerulus (glomerular filtration). As the filtrate passes down the nephron and through the tubules its volume is reduced and water and solutes are removed (tubular reabsorption) and waste products are secreted (tubular secretion).

(b) A nephron consists of an individual renal tubule and its glomerulus. Each tubule has several segments, beginning with the proximal tubule, followed by the loop of Henle (descending and ascending limbs), the distal convoluted tubule, the connecting tubule, and the collecting duct.

(c) The kidneys receive just under 25% of the cardiac output.

(d) Renal blood flow enters the glomerulus via the afferent arteriole and leaves via the efferent arteriole (whose diameter is smaller). Renal blood flow is regulated by norepinephrine (constriction, reduction of flow), dopamine (vasodilation, increases flow), angiotensin II (constricts), prostaglandins (dilation in the renal cortex and constriction in the renal medulla), and acetylcholine (vasodilation).

(e) Urine is stored in the bladder before voiding (micturition). The micturition response involves reflex pathways, but is under voluntary control.

(f) Total body osmolality is directly proportional to the total body sodium plus the total body potassium divided by the total body water. Changes in the osmolality of the body fluids occur when a disproportion exists between the amount of these electrolytes and the amount of water ingested or lost from the body.

(g) The amount of Na^+ in the ECF is the most important determinant of ECF volume, and mechanisms that control Na^+ balance are the major mechanisms defending ECF volume. The main mechanism regulating sodium balance is the renin–angiotensin system, a hormone system that regulates blood pressure.

(h) The kidneys secrete the enzyme renin and renin acts in concert with angiotensin-converting enzyme to form angiotensin II. Angiotensin II acts directly on the adrenal cortex to increase the secretion of aldosterone. Aldosterone increases the retention of sodium from the urine via action on the renal collecting duct.

(i) The cells of the proximal and distal tubules secrete hydrogen ions. Acidification also occurs in the collecting ducts. The reaction that is primarily responsible for H^+ secretion in the proximal tubules is Na^+–H^+ exchange. Na is absorbed from the lumen of the tubule and H is excreted.

(j) Three important reactions in the tubular fluid remove free H^+, permitting more acid to be secreted. These are the reactions with HCO_3^- to form CO_2 and H_2O, with HPO_4^{2-} to form $H_2PO_4^-$, and with NH_3 to form NH_4^+.

(k) The composition of urine- 93% to 97% water, urea, creatinine, ammonia, uric acid, urobilin, and bilirubin, sodium, chloride, potassium, sulphate, magnesium, calcium and other ions.

Questions

1. Define urinary system.
2. Enlist components of urinary system
3. Draw the figure of urinary system
4. What is kidney?
5. What is ACE?

***

Experiment No. 16

Aim: To study the structure and functions of reproductive system.

Basis of Genetic Sex:

The differences between the two sexes depend on the presence of a single chromosome the Y chromosome and two endocrine structures, the testis and the ovaries. The hormonal secretions from the testis are responsible for the development of the male external genitalia and male sexual behaviour. The sex of the individual is determined genetically by two chromosomes (X and Y), called the sex chromosomes. Each individual has two sex chromosomes XX (female) or XY (male) and 22 other pairs of chromosomes, called autosomes. When the ovaries in the mother and the testis in the father manufacture reproductive cells (the ova and sperm, respectively), only one of the sex chromosomes is present in each of the cells. This is because cell division occurs by meiosis. Each ovum from the female contains one X chromosome (in addition to 22 autosomes). Of the sperm, some contain one Y chromosome and others contain one X chromosome (in addition to 22 autosomes). Therefore, when the ova and sperm come together during fertilization, two types of combinations can occur XX (genetic female) and XY (genetic male). The fertilized ovum has 23 pairs of chromosomes (22 autosomes plus two sex chromosomes).

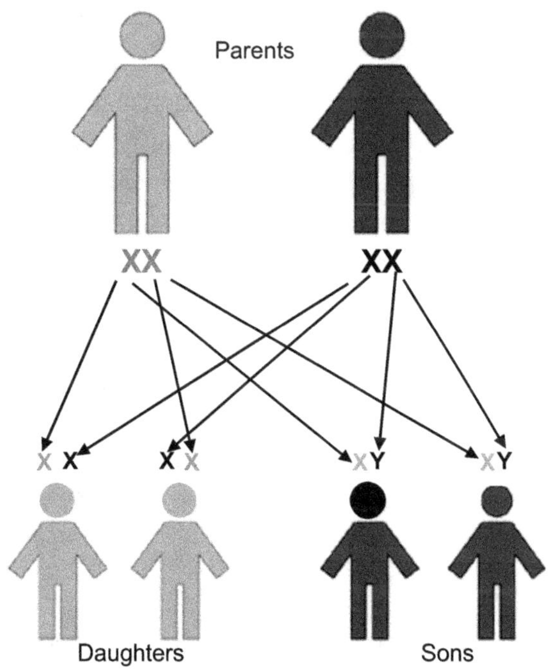

Fig. 16.1: Reproductive System

The Male Reproductive System:

The male reproductive system consists of the gonads (testis) that produce gametes and hormones; the ducts that receive and transport the gametes; the accessory glands that secrete fluid into the ducts for the nourishment and maintenance of the gametes; and the external structures associated with the reproductive system, collectively known as the external genitalia.

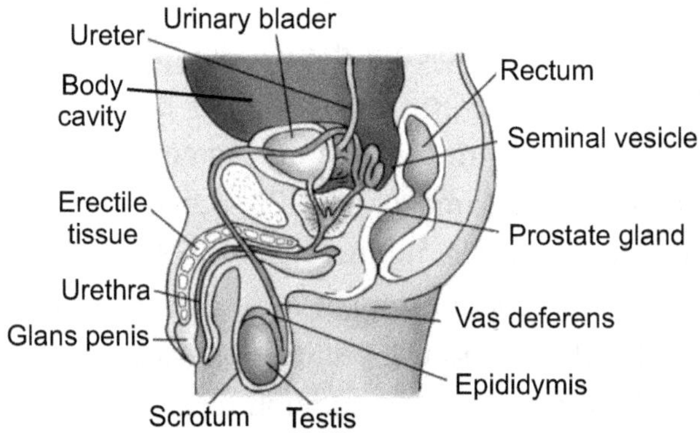

Fig. 16.2: Male reproductive system

The Testis:

Each testis, shaped like a flattened egg, is about 5 cm long, 3 cm wide, and 2.5 cm thick. The testis hangs inside the scrotum a pouch that lies posterior to the penis and anterior to the anus. In the fetus, the testis develops inside the abdominal cavity close to the kidney.

The Scrotum:

The scrotum consists of a thin layer of skin and underlying fascia. The fascia has a layer of smooth muscle known as dartos, which is responsible for the wrinkles seen in the skin. Deep to the dermis, there is a layer of skeletal muscle known as the cremaster muscle. The contraction of this muscle causes the testis to be pulled closer to the body when cold. Relaxation of the muscle causes the testis to move away from the body. Thus, the temperature of the testis is maintained about 1.1°C (34°F) below that of the body—the temperature required for normal sperm production. Internally, the scrotum is divided into two chambers. A testis lies in each of these chambers or cavities. The testis is separated from the inner surface of the scrotum by a space lined by serous membrane. The membrane, known as the tunica vaginalis, is a remnant of the peritoneum through which the testis pushed during development. The tunica vaginalis reduces the friction between the testis and the scrotum.

The Mature Sperm (Spermatozoa):

Each sperm has a rounded head and a long tail. The head houses the nucleus with densely packed chromosomes. The head is covered by a cap (acrosomal cap), which contains the enzymes required for digesting the outer layer of the ova at the time of fertilization. The long tail helps the sperm propel forward with a rapid, corkscrew motion. Because the sperm does not have energy reserves, it relies on the surrounding fluid for survival.

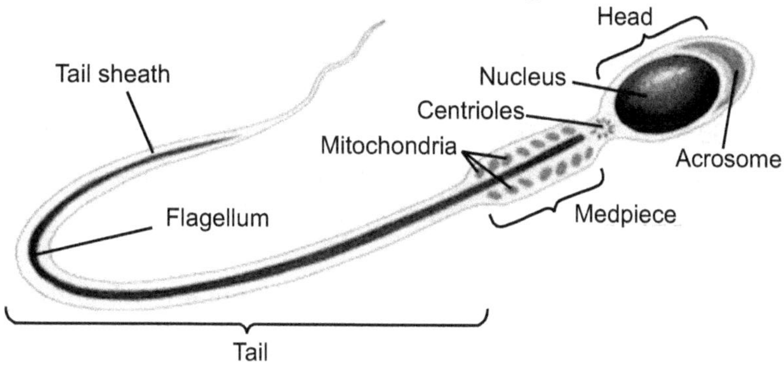

Fig. 16.3: Sperm

Epididymis:

The seminiferous tubules drain into a network of ducts, which, in turn, are continuous with a highly coiled structure known as the epididymis. The epididymis lies along the posterior border of the testis and consists of a coiled tubule about 7 meters long. This tubule continues as the vas deferens or ductus deferens from the inferior portion of the testis. It also removes damaged sperm and dead cells. In addition, it stores the sperm and facilitates its maturation. The sperm are moved along the reproductive tract by peristaltic contractions of the smooth muscle in the walls of the tubule.

Vas Deferens:

The vas deferens is a tube about 45 cm long. It begins at the inferior, posterior aspect of the testis and ascends superiorly and enters the inguinal canal. The vas deferens, together with the blood vessels, lymphatic vessels, nerves, muscles, and connective tissue fascia that surrounds it in this region, is known as the spermatic cord. It extends from the deep and inferior aspect of the anterior abdominal wall the deep inguinal ring to the testis. The structures, after entering the deep inguinal ring, pass through the inguinal canal, exit through the superficial inguinal ring, and descend superficially to reach the testis. At this point, the vas deferens enlarges slightly to form the ampulla. The duct from the accessory gland (seminal vesicle) joins it here to form the ejaculatory duct. This duct passes through the prostate gland and empties into the prostatic urethra. The urethra extends from the urinary bladder to the tip of the penis. It is about 20 cm long and passes through the prostate (prostatic urethra), connective tissue in the perineum (membranous urethra), and the penis (penile urethra).

Accessory Glands:

The seminal vesicle, together with the prostate and bulbourethral gland, form the accessory glands. These glands function to provide the nutrients required by the sperm for motility, to activate the sperm, to help propel the sperm along the reproductive tract, and to counteract the acidity of the urethral and vaginal contents. The secretions of the glands and the contraction of smooth muscles are regulated by the autonomic nervous system.

Seminal Vesicles:

The two seminal vesicles are located on the posterior aspect of the urinary bladder, embedded in the connective tissue between the bladder and the rectum. The two glands contribute about 60% of the semen fluid. The fluid contains fructose (nutrient), prostaglandins (stimulates contraction of smooth muscles), and fibrinogen (which helps the fluid to form a temporary clot in the vagina), among other substances.

Prostate Gland:

The prostate gland is a muscular, rounded organ of about 4 cm. It surrounds the urethra as it leaves the bladder and consists of 30 to 50 compound tubule alveolar glands that open into the urethra. The fluid secreted by the prostate is acidic and contains, among others, an antibiotic that prevents urinary tract infection. Its secretion makes up 25% of the voume of semen.

The Bulbourethral Glands:

The two bulbourethral glands (Cowper's glands) are situated at the base of the penis. They secrete thick, alkaline mucus, which helps to neutralize the acidity and provide lubrication.

Semen:

During ejaculation, the propulsion of sperm from the urethra to the exterior, about 2–5 mL of semen (ejaculate) is expelled. Each milliliter of ejaculate contains about 20–100 million sperm/milliliter. The fluid from the seminiferous tubules contributes 5% of the semen, and the accessory glands provide the rest. Thus, the fluid component of the semen is a mixture of secretions from the seminiferous tubule and the accessory glands.

Penis:

The penis is the tubular organ through which the urethra passes before it opens into the exterior. The penile urethra serves as a common passage for urine as well as ejaculate. The penis helps to introduce the ejaculate into the vagina of the female. The penis consists of a maze of vascular channels in three cylindrical columns two corpus cavernosa and one corpus spongiosum. The columns are surrounded by thick, elastic connective tissue and smooth muscle. The blood flow through the channels varies according to the state of sexual arousal. The penis is divided into the root, body, neck, and glans. The root is the portion attached to the body wall, inferior to the pubic symphysis, and consists of the bulb of the penis (the expanded portion of the corpora spongiosum) and the crura (the two, separated portions of the corpora cavernosa). The bulb of the penis is attached to the perineal muscles and fascia and is surrounded by the skeletal muscle (bulbospongiosus). The body (shaft) is the movable portion and the glans is the enlarged distal end. The neck is the narrow portion between the shaft and the glans. The thin, delicate fold of skin that overlies the tip of the penis is known as the prepuce.

Endocrine Function of the Testis:

The male sex hormones are known as androgens. The major hormone secreted by the interstitial cells (Leydig cells) of the testis is testosterone. Testosterone is a steroid hormone and, like all steroids, is derived from cholesterol. The adrenal cortex also contributes to the concentration of androgens in the plasma. At the time of fetal development, as mentioned, testosterone has an effect on the brain, resulting in the male pattern of behaviour. It also stimulates the development of the internal male genitalia. Later, testosterone develops and maintains the male secondary sex characteristics. It also has a growth-promoting and protein-building effect.

Control of Testosterone Secretion:

Testosterone secretion is controlled by follicular stimulating hormone (FSH) and luteinizing hormone (LH) from the anterior pituitary. FSH and LH are, in turn, controlled by gonadotropin releasing hormone (GnRH) secreted by the hypothalamus. FSH is required for sperm manufacture. LH mainly functions to stimulate production of testosterone. The level of testosterone in the plasma has a negative feedback effect on the hypothalamus and pituitary. The cells of the testis also produce another hormone known as inhibin, which helps to regulate the secretion of FSH.

The Female Reproductive System:

The function of the female reproductive system is to produce sex hormones, functioning gametes (ova), and to support and protect the developing embryo. The major organs are the ovaries (gonads), uterine tubes (fallopian tubes or oviducts), the uterus, the vagina, accessory glands, and the components of the external genitalia. The breasts (mammary glands) are also considered part of the female reproductive system.

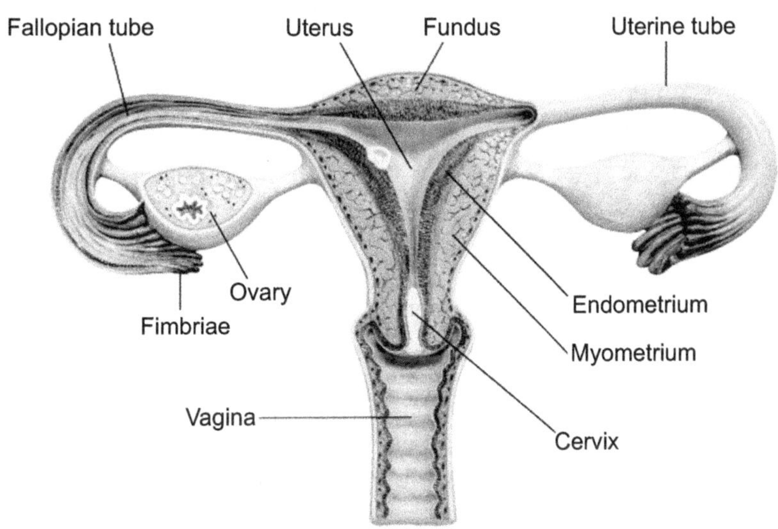

Fig. 16.4: Female reproductive system

The Ovaries:

The two ovaries are almond-shaped organs, about 5 cm long, 2.5 cm wide and 8 mm thick, located near the lateral walls of the pelvic cavity. The ovaries are held in place by ligaments that connect them to the uterus (ovarian ligament) and the pelvis (suspensory ligament). The surface of the ovary is nodular and has ova (primordial follicle) in various stages of development. At the time of birth, there are about 2 million immature ova in the ovaries. Many of the ova degenerate; at puberty, there are only about 400,000 remaining. The immature ova (oocytes) lie dormant in the ovary until they are stimulated by a sudden surge in the hormone FSH at puberty. Every month thereafter, some of the oocytes undergo further development. This is known as the ovarian cycle.

Uterine Tubes (Fallopian Tubes; Oviduct):

Each muscular uterine tube is about 12 cm long. One end is free and opens into the pelvic cavity and the other end is continuous, with the superior and lateral aspect of the uterus. The free end of the tube, the infundibulum, is expanded and funnel shaped, with fingerlike projections known as fimbriae. The fimbriae are in close contact with the ovary, especially at ovulation. The fallopian tube is lined with ciliated epithelium, which help move the ovum toward the uterine cavity.

The Uterus:

The non-pregnant uterus is a pear shaped organ about 7.5 cm long and 5 cm wide (at the widest diameter). It lies suspended between the urinary bladder anteriorly and the rectum posteriorly. The upper portion of the uterus is normally bent forward, lying over the superior and posterior aspect of the urinary bladder. Part of the superior portion of the uterus is covered by the peritoneum. The uterus can be divided into the anatomic regions the body and the cervix. The body is the largest region of the uterus. The part of the body of the uterus above the attachment of the uterine tubes is known as the fundus. Inferiorly, the body becomes narrower and continues down as the cervix. The cervix is the region of the uterus that projects into the vagina.

The Uterine Walls:

The uterus has a thick, muscular wall, consisting of three layers. The outer layer is the perimetrium, which is actually part of the peritoneum covering the superior aspect. Deep to the perimetrium is the muscular myometrium. The third and innermost layer is the endometrium, a glandular mucosa lining the uterine cavity. The myometrium consists of smooth muscle arranged in longitudinal, oblique, and circular layers. It forms 90% of the uterine wall and is responsible for the powerful contractions that occur at the time of labour. The endometrium is the inner lining that undergoes cyclical changes influenced by hormones. It has an abundant blood supply and numerous glands that help support the growing fetus at the time of pregnancy.

The Uterine Cavity:

The uterine cavity is somewhat triangular in shape, with the base of the triangle located superiorly. The openings of the fallopian tubes are located in the two upper angles. The lower end of the cavity narrows to a portion known as the uterine isthmus. The isthmus is continuous with the opening of the cervix, which projects about 1.5 cm into the vagina. The passage in the middle of the cervix is known as the cervical canal. The two ends of the cervical canal are known as the internal (opens into the uterine cavity) and external os (opens into the vagina).

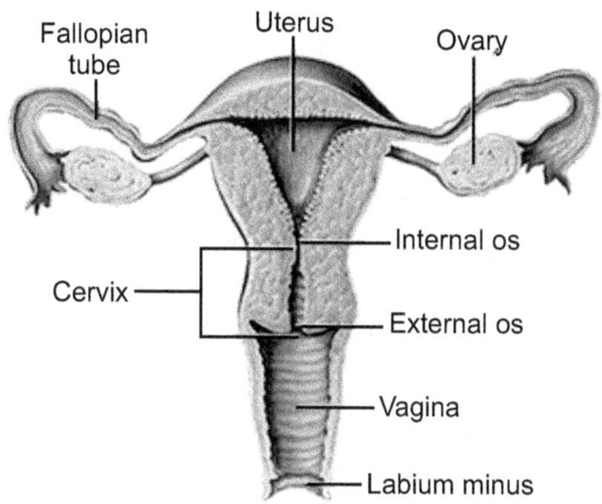

Fig. 16.5: Uterine cavity

Uterine Support:

The ovaries, uterine tubes and the uterus are held in place inside the abdomen by ligaments that connect them to the surrounding walls. Laterally, the peritoneum covers the fallopian tube and becomes continuous with the walls of the pelvis. The sheet of peritoneum lateral to the uterus is known as the broad ligament and serves to support the uterus. Another pair of ligaments the uterosacral ligament runs from the lateral surface of the uterus to the anterior aspect of the sacrum, holding the uterus in place and preventing it from sliding anteriorly and inferiorly. The round ligaments run from the lateral aspect of the uterus, just below the uterine tube toward the lateral wall of the pelvis into the inguinal canal, preventing the uterus from sliding posteriorly. Another pair of ligaments, the lateral ligaments, runs from the lower end of the uterus near the vagina to the lateral wall of the pelvis, preventing inferior movement of the uterus. The skeletal muscles and the fascia covering the pelvic outlet further help support the uterus.

The Vagina:

The vagina is a muscular, extensible elastic tube about 10 cm long, which extends from the cervix to the external genitalia. The cervix protrudes into the vagina. The part of the vagina surrounding the cervix is the fornix. In women who have not had intercourse, a thin epithelial fold the hymen partially or fully covers the opening of the vagina. Skeletal muscles similar to that present in the male, the bulbospongiosus, extend along the sides of the vagina and help constrict the opening. The vagina is lined by stratified squamous epithelium and houses many harmless bacteria, whose acidic secretions prevent harmful organisms from thriving there.

The Perineum:

The perineum denotes the region between the thighs and buttocks that houses the external genitalia and anus in both sexes. The perineum extends to the pubic symphysis anteriorly, to the ischialtuberosities laterally, and to the coccyx posteriorly.

Menstrual Cycle:

After puberty, the female reproductive system, unlike that of the male, undergoes cyclical changes that can be regarded as periodic preparation for fertilization and pregnancy. This cyclical change is known as the menstrual cycle. The most conspicuous of these changes is the vaginal bleeding that occurs with the shedding of part of the inner lining of the uterus (menstruation). The duration of the cycle is variable. Typically, the cycle lasts for 28 days, with day 1 denoted as the first day of menstruation and day 28 as the day before menstruation of the next cycle. Although the menstrual cycle has effects throughout the body, only those changes occurring in the ovary, fallopian tube, uterus, vagina, and breast are described here. The changes in the cycle are a result of the ebb and surge of sex hormone levels in the plasma.

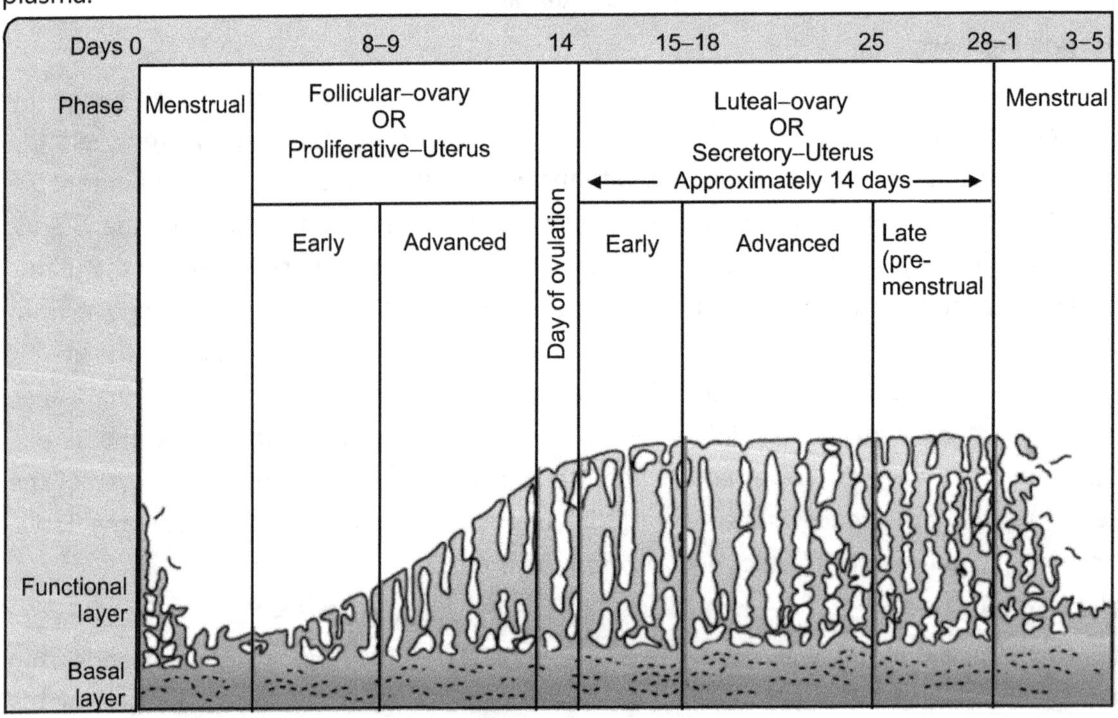

Fig. 16.6: Menstrual cycle

Ovarian Cycle and Fate of the Ova:

At the beginning of every cycle, a cavity filled with fluid forms around the oocytes (primordial follicles) in the ovary. Soon, one of the follicles rapidly increases in size while the others regress. This is the dominant follicle. Certain cells in the follicle secrete the hormone estrogen. About 14 days before the start of the next cycle, the enlarged follicle ruptures and the ovum is extruded into the abdominal cavity. This process is known as ovulation. The ovum is picked up by the fimbriae of the uterine tubes and transported into the uterus. If fertilization occurs, the fertilized ovum embeds in the uterine cavity wall. If unfertilized, it is expelled from the uterus into the vagina and then outside the body at the time of menstruation. After ovulation, the ruptured follicle in the ovary fills up with blood. The cells lining the follicle rapidly multiply and yellowish, lipid-rich cells known as the luteal cells replace the clotted blood. The follicle is now known as the corpus luteum. The luteal cells secrete the hormones estrogens and progesterone. If pregnancy occurs, the corpus luteum persists and menstruation does not occur until delivery as a result of continuous estrogen and progesterone secretion. If there is no pregnancy, the corpus luteum degenerates by about 12 days after ovulation and is eventually replaced by scar tissue. The phase from the 1st day of menstruation to the day of ovulation is known as the follicular or preovulatory phase. Since follicular enlargement is brought about by estrogen secretion, this phase is also known as the estrogenic phase. After ovulation, as the remnants of the follicle are replaced by luteal cells, the rest of the menstrual cycle is known as the luteal phase. This phase is also known as the progestational phase because of the high level of progesterone at this time.

Changes in the Uterus:

At the beginning of the menstrual cycle, the uterine cavity has only the remnants of the deep layer of the endometrium. From the fifth to the fourteenth days, the endometrium rapidly increases in thickness, and the uterine glands lengthen. This phase of the cycle is referred to as the proliferative phase. After ovulation, the endometrium becomes highly vascularized. The glands coil and secrete a clear fluid. Hence, this phase (from the 14 to 28 days) is known as the secretory phase. If the ovum is not fertilized, the endometrium becomes thinner and areas of cell death (necrosis) begin to appear in the endometrium. Blood vessels go into spasm and some bleeding is seen. The inner lining of the endometrium sloughs off and this collection of dead cells, together with the blood, is the menstrual flow.

Normal Menstruation:

Normally, the menstrual blood contains 75% arterial and 25% venous blood. It contains tissue debris from the endometrial lining together with prostaglandin and fibrinolysin (an enzyme that prevents clotting); therefore, clots are not seen in the menstrual flow. Usually, menstruation lasts from 3-5 days (range, 1-8 days). Functionally, the uterus restores the endometrium from the previous menstruation during the proliferative phase and prepares to embed the fertilized ovum during the secretory phase. The length of the secretory phase is remarkably constant at 14 days from the day of ovulation to the beginning of the next menstrual cycle.

Changes in the Cervix:

The cervical mucosa and its secretions also undergo cyclical changes. The mucus secreted is thinner (less viscous) and more alkaline during the follicular phase. These changes promote survival and motility of the sperm. During the secretory or luteal phase, the secretions become thicker.

Changes in the Vagina:

The cells in the vagina also undergo cyclical changes. During the later part of the cycle, the epithelium becomes thicker and is infiltrated with white blood cells. The mucus secretion becomes thicker during this phase.

Changes in the Breast:

During the proliferative phase, the ducts of the mammary gland increase in number and size. In the later half of the cycle, the lobules of the glands increase in size. The blood flow is increased and fluid tends to accumulate in the interstitial tissue. This is responsible for the tenderness, swelling, and pain experienced by individuals about 10 days before the start of the next cycle. All of these symptoms disappear at the start of menstruation.

Changes in Body Temperature:

In addition to the previously mentioned changes, the basal body temperature also fluctuates. At the time of ovulation, the temperature (taken orally or rectally in the morning before rising from bed) is raised by about 0.5°C (32.9°F). This, along with other cyclical changes, can be used to determine the time of ovulation.

Menstrual Cycle Regulation:

All changes that occur during the menstrual cycles are a result of the changing levels of hormones secreted by the hypothalamus, pituitary, and ovaries.

***The Role of the Hypothalamus*:**

The hormones secreted by the pituitary are controlled by gonadotropin-releasing hormone (GnRH) of the hypothalamus. Because of the connections of the hypothalamus with the rest of the nervous system, hormones secreted by it can be altered according to changes detected by the nervous system in the external environment.

The Role of the Pituitary Gland:

The pituitary secretes two hormones, follicle-stimulating hormone (FSH) and luteinizing hormone (LH). FSH stimulates the growth of ovarian follicles. LH is responsible for the final maturation of the follicles and estrogen secretion from the ovary. A sudden increase in levels of plasma LH results in ovulation. LH also causes the development of the ruptured ovarian follicle into the corpus luteum (in the later part of the cycle) and secretion of the hormones estrogen and progesterone by the corpus luteum.

The Role of the Ovaries:

As previously mentioned, the ovaries secrete the female sex hormones estrogen and progesterone. The secretion of estrogen peaks twice during the menstrual cycle; once just before ovulation and once in the middle of the luteal phase.

Estrogen:

The hormone estrogen affects many organs. It facilitates the growth of the ovarian follicle and increases the motility of the fallopian tubes. It increases the size of the uterus and excitability of the uterine smooth muscles. It also sensitizes the uterus to the hormone oxytocin at the time of labour. Estrogen accelerates the growth of long bones and closure of epiphysis at puberty and decreases the rate of bone resorption. Estrogens tend to lower the levels of cholesterol in the blood. This may be one of the reasons for the lower incidence of cardiovascular disease, such as atherosclerosis, in women.

Progesterone:

Progesterone is a hormone secreted mainly by the corpus luteum. The primordial follicles also secrete small amounts. During pregnancy, the placenta secretes this hormone. The principal organs affected by this hormone are the brain, uterus, and breasts. It is responsible for the cyclical changes that occur in the luteal phase of the menstrual cycle and for the slight increase in body temperature at the time of ovulation.

Relaxin:

The ovaries secrete a hormone called relaxin. This hormone is also secreted by the placenta in pregnant women. Relaxin relaxes the pubic symphysis and other pelvic joints and softens and dilates the uterine cervix at the time of pregnancy.

Questions

1. Give principal of reproductive system.
2. Explain male reproductive system.
3. Explain female reproductive system.
4. Draw the figure of sperm.
5. Comment on vagina.

***

Experiment No. 17

Aim: To study family planning devices and pregnancy diagnosis test.

Requirements:

1. Family planning kit.

Theory:

Family planning refers to attain certain objectives like:

1. To avoid unwanted births.
2. To bring about wanted births.
3. To regulate intervals between pregnancies.
4. To control the time at which birth occurs in relation to the ages of the parent and
5. To determine the number of children in the family.

Devices for family planning: The measures for family planning include various contraceptive methods that regulate the fertility and control child birth.

Contraceptive methods: These are defined as the preventive methods that help women to avoid unwanted pregnancies.

Though many contraceptive methods have been available there can never be an ideal contraceptive which will be safe, effective, acceptable, inexpensive, reversible, simple to administer, long lasting, and with little or no medical supervision. Also a method which may be quite suitable for one group may be unsuitable for other because of difference in cultural pattern, religious belief and socioeconomic status. As there is no any single method to meet need of individual as well as community family planning programmes offer all the methods from which individual can choose according to his need and wish.

The term conventional contraceptives is used to denote the methods that require action at the time to sexual intercourse. e.g. condoms, spermicides etc. Each contraceptive method has its own advantages or disadvantages and the success of contraceptive method depends on its effectiveness in preventing pregnancy as well as the rate of continuation of its proper use.

The contraceptive methods are mainly classified into two types: (a) Spacing methods and (b) Terminal methods.

(a) Spacing methods:

1. Barrier methods
   (a) Physical methods
   (b) Chemical methods
   (c) Combined methods

2. Intra-uterine devices
3. Hormonal methods
4. Post-conceptional methods
5. Miscellaneous
   (a) Terminal methods
      1. Male sterilization
      2. Female sterilization

(a) Spacing methods:

(1) Barrier methods: Number of barrier methods or occlusive methods are available for men as well as women. These methods prevent the fertilization of ovum by the sperm. These methods offer certain contraceptive as well as non-contraceptive advantages. The contraceptive advantage includes absence of side effect which commonly occurs with pills or IUDs. The non-contraceptive advantages are some protection against sexually transmitted diseases (STDs) and reduction in risk of cervical cancer. They are less effective than pill or the loop. They are effective only if used consistently and carefully.

(a) Physical methods: It includes use of some physical barrier that prevents entry of sperm in cervix. It includes condoms, diaphragms and vaginal sponge.

(i) Condom: It is most widely known and used barrier device as it has less side effects and prevent transmission of STDs in both men and women. The condom is fitted on the erect penis before intercourse. A new condom should be used for each sexual act.

Advantages of condom:

1. Easily available, safe and inexpensive.
2. Easy to use as do not need medical supervision.
3. No side effects.
4. Light, compact and disposable.
5. Provide protection against pregnancy as well as STDs.

Disadvantages:

(a) It may slip off or tear if used incorrectly and

(b) Some men may complain about lack of sexual sensation and many men do not use it though the risk of pregnancy and STD is high.

(ii) Diaphragm: It is a vaginal barrier invented by German physician in 1882. It is also known as "Dutch cap". It is a shallow cup made of synthetic rubber or plastic material with flexible rim of spring or metal. It is inserted into vagina before sexual intercourse and must remain in place for at least hours after intercourse. A spermicidal jelly is always used along with it. The cervical cap, vault cap, vimule cap are the some variations in the diaphragm but these devices are not recommended by National Family Planning Programme.

Advantages:

The advantages of diaphragm are total absence of risks and no any medical contraindication.

Disadvantage:

Initially demonstration of technique for its insertion by physician or technical person is needed. A proper muscle tone of vaginal muscles is required to hold the diaphragm in position. They must be removed and washed properly after intercourse. If it left in vagina for longer time produces toxic shock syndrome due to bacterial infections of upper part of vagina.

(iii) Vaginal Sponge: The use of sponge soaked in vinegar or olive oil is the ancient method of contraception. Now it is marketed in USA under the trade name "Today" which consist of small polyurethane foam sponge saturated with spermicidal nonoxynol-9. It is less effective device.

(b) Chemical Methods: The use of certain spermicidal for contraception is known as chemical method. These include four categories

Foams: Foam tablets, foam aerosols.

Creams, jellies and pastes: Squeezed from tube.

Suppositories: Inserted manually.

Soluble films: C-film inserted manually.

Disadvantages of Spermicides are:

(i) High failure rate.

(ii) Must be used immediately before intercourse and repeated use of each sexual act.

(iii) Must be introduced in the vagina in region where sperms are like to be deposited.

(iv) May cause mild burning and irritation.

The use of chemical methods is not that much recommended due to safety concern.

(2) Intrauterine devices: The device which is inserted in uterus to prevent conception is known as Intrauterine device (IUD). The concept of insertion of some foreign body in to the uterus and prevention of conception is the old concept known to human beings. The first original device that was used as intrauterine device was silkworm gut in 1909. In 1929 Grafenburgh, a German Gynaecologist used IUD made of silver successfully. The IUDs are made of polyethylene or other polymers.

Types of IUD:

Two types of IUDs are:

1. Non-medicated.
2. Medicated

The non-medicated IUDs also known as inert IUDs are often referred as first generation IUDs. They are available in various shapes and sizes- loops, spirals, coils, rings and bows.

The IUDs comprising copper are referred as Second generation IUDs. It was found that metallic copper had a strong anti fertility effect so copper was added to IUDs. These are also available in various sizes and shapes e.g. Copper-7, Copper T-200, T Cu-220 C. The number included in the name refers to the surface area of the copper on the device.

Copper IUDs primarily work by disrupting sperm mobility and damaging sperm so that they are prevented from joining with an ovum. Copper acts as a spermicide within the uterus, increasing levels of copper ions, prostaglandins, and white blood cells within the uterine and tubal fluids. The increased copper ions in the cervical mucus inhibit the sperm's motility and viability, preventing sperm from traveling through the cervical mucus or destroying it as it passes through. Copper IUDs have a first year failure rate ranging from 0.1 to 2.2%.

The Copper IUDs containing noble metals are becoming increasingly popular because they are more resistant to corrosion. So the copper IUDs with gold, silver and combination of silver and gold are prepared and used in some countries.

The hormone releasing IUDs are known as Third generation IUDs. These IUDs release a hormone. The most widely used hormonal device is progestasert which is a T-shaped device filled with progesterone. The hormone is released slowly in the uterus at a rate 65 mcg daily. The hormone produces local effect on the uterine lining, on the cervical mucus and on the sperms. It increases the viscosity of the cervical mucus and prevents entry of sperm into cervix. It also makes the endometrium unfavourable for the implantation of fertilized ovum.

Advantages of IUDs:

1. Simple method of insertion, no hospitalization is required.
2. Insertion takes only few minutes.
3. Once inserted IUD remains in place as long as required.
4. Inexpensive.
5. Contraceptive effect is reversible after removal of IUD.
6. No systemic-metabolic side effects.
7. Some side effects and complications may occur with use of IUDs. They are:

Disadvantages:

1. Increased vaginal bleeding.
2. Pain.
3. Pelvic infection.
4. Uterine perforation.
5. Ectopic pregnancy.

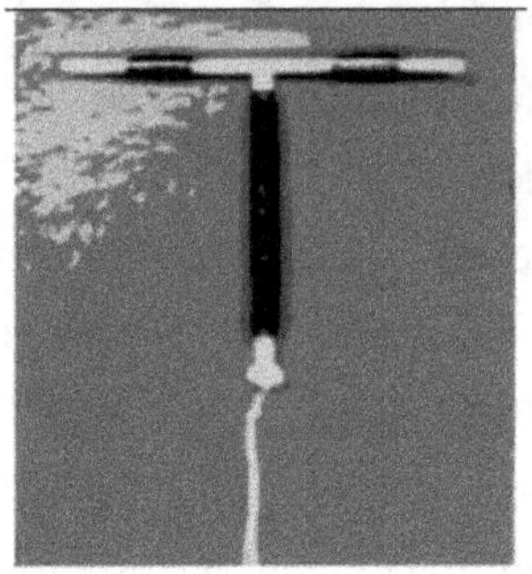	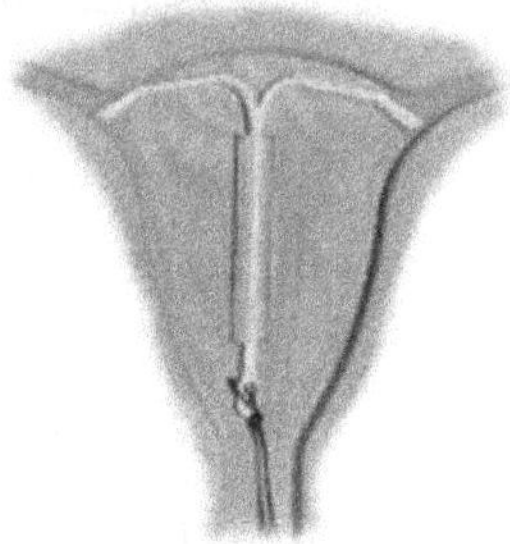	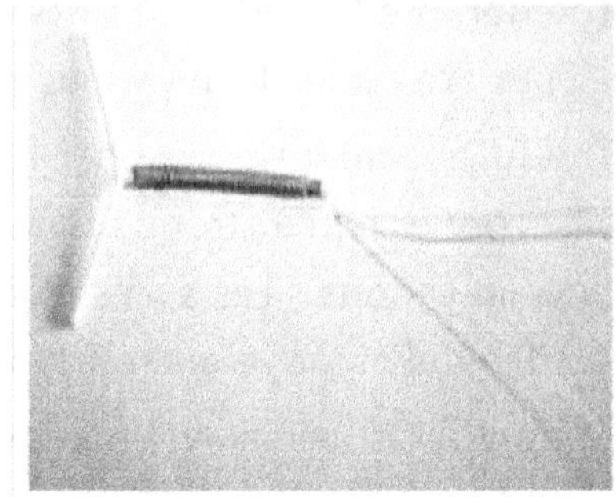
Copper-T	Harmonal IUD	Copper T with string

Fig. 17.1: Intrauterine devices

(3) Hormonal method:

Hormonal contraception refers to method that acts on the endocrine system. Almost all hormonal methods are composed of steroid hormones. The original hormonal method the combined oral contraceptive pill was first marketed as a contraceptive in 1960. Altogether, 18% of the world's contraceptive users rely on hormonal methods. Hormonal contraception is highly effective: when taken on the prescribed schedule, users of steroid hormone methods experience pregnancy rates of less than 1% per year. Perfect-use pregnancy rates for most hormonal contraceptives are usually around the 0.3% rate or less. Currently available methods can only be used by women. The development of a male hormonal contraceptive is an active research area. The hormonal contraceptives act by inhibition of ovulation and inhibiting entry of sperm in the uterus by thickening of the cervical mucus.

The hormonal contraceptives are classified as follows:

(A) Oral pills:

1. Combined pills.
2. Progestogen-only pill (POP).
3. Post coital pill.
4. Once a month (long acting) pill.
5. Male pill.

(B) Depot (Slow release) Formulation:

1. Injectables.
2. Subcutaneous implants.
3. Vaginal rings.

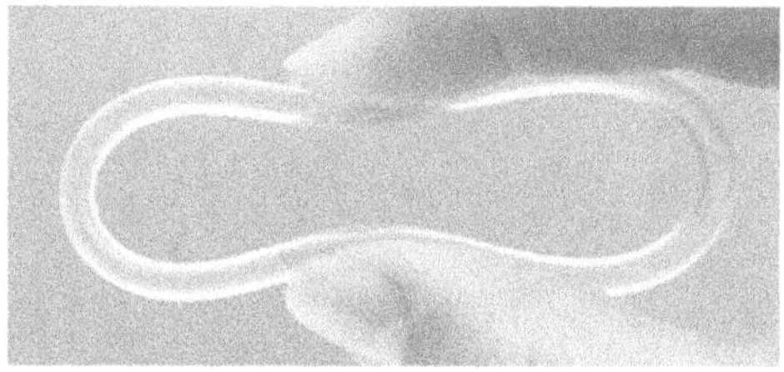

Fig. 17.2: Oral Pills

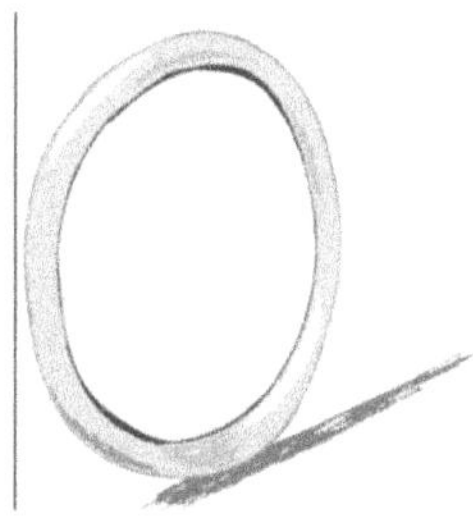

Fig. 17.3: Vaginal rings

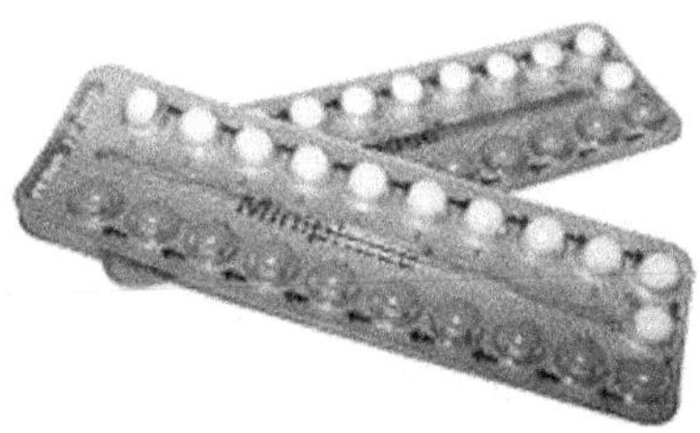

Fig. 17.4: Combined pill

Combined Pill: The most popular form of hormonal contraception, the combined oral contraceptive pill is known commonly as the pill. It is taken once a day, most commonly for 21 days followed by a seven-day break, although other regimens are also used. Govt. of India has made available 2 types of low dose oral pills under the brand names of MALA-N, and MALA-D.

Progestogen-only pill (POP): It is commonly referred to as minipill or micropill. It contains only progestogen which is given in small doses throughout the cycle. The commonly used progestogens are norethisterone and levonorgestrel.

Post coital pill: Post coital contraception is recommended within 48 hours of an unprotected intercourse. A very high dose of an estrogen (diethyl-stilbosterol) is used in high dose.

Still a promising long acting pill and male pill is not available. A research on this is still going on.

Advantages of oral pills:

1. Effective.
2. Cost effective.
3. Increased acceptance.

Provide non-contraceptive advantages to treat some medical conditions as polycystic ovary syndrome (PCOS), endometriosis, amenorrhea, menstrual cramps, adenomyosis, menorrhagia (excessive menstral bleeding), menstruation-related anemia and dysmenorrhea (painful menstruation).

Disadvantages:

1. Need the medical supervision.
2. Interaction with other drugs.
3. Systemic metabolic abnormalities can be produced.
4. Serious side effects such as carcinogenesis, cardiovascular disorders, liver disorders.

(B) Depot formulation:

The depot formulation of hormones are highly effective, reversible, long acting and estrogen free and single dose administration contraceptives.

(i) Injectable contraceptives: Two progestogen have been found suitable as contraceptives. They are DMPA (Depot medroxyprogesterone acetate) and NET-EN (Norethisterone enantate). The initial injection of both should be given during the first 5 days of the menstrual period as intramuscular injection. Both the hormones have side effects as disruption of the normal menstrual cycle, intermittent bleeding etc.

(ii) Subdermal implants: A contraceptive implant is a birth control device inserted under the skin by a doctor. The implant is among the most effective birth control methods. After it is inserted it prevents pregnancy by releasing hormones that prevent ovulation and prevent entry of sperm into cervix by thickening cervical mucous. The implant can prevent pregnancy for up to three years. Though it protects against pregnancy, it does not protect against STIs. Norplant, Implanon, Sino- Implan are some brands available. Norplant consist of 6 silicone rubber capsules each containing 35 mg of levonorgesterol.

Advantages:

1. It does not interrupt sexual satisfaction.
2. Women have fewer, lighter periods.
3. 30% Women have no more bleeding periods (sign of total efficacity).
4. Lasts for up to 3 years (less if overweight).
5. Can be used while breastfeeding.
6. May lessen typical premenstrual symptoms.

Disadvantages:

1. Irregular bleeding for the first 6–12 months.
2. Less common: Change in appetite, depression, headache, nausea, nervousness, sore breasts.
3. Weight gain, dizziness, pregnancy symptoms, hair loss, facial hair gain, lethargic feeling.

(iii) Vaginal rings: Vaginal rings containing levonorgesterol have been found to be effective. The hormone is slowly absorbed through the vaginal mucosa and bypass digestive system and liver. The ring is worn in the vagina for 3 weeks of the cycle and removed in the fourth.

(4) Post-Conceptional method: These methods include termination of pregnancy. These methods are menstrual regulation, menstrual induction and abortion.

The menstrual regulation consists of aspiration of the uterine contents 6-14 days of missed period but before that the pregnancy by suitable test must be confirmed. Menstrual induction includes disturbing the normal progesterone- prostaglandin balance by intrauterine application of 1-5 mg of prostaglandin F_2. Within few minutes of application of prostaglandin the contraction starts and bleeding starts which continues upto 7-8 days. Abortion is theoretically determined as termination of pregnancy before the foetus becomes viable i.e. capable of living independently.

(5) Miscellaneous methods: These methods include complete absence to sexual activity, interruption of coitus (thereby the deposition of semen in vagina is prevented), safe period method, natural family planning methods.

(a) Terminal methods: The terminal methods includes male and female sterilization.

(i) Male sterilization: Vasectomy is a surgical procedure for male sterilization and/or permanent birth control. During the procedure, the vasa deferentia of a man are cut off, and then tied/sealed in a manner such to prevent sperm from entering into the seminal stream (ejaculate). Vasectomies are usually performed in by physicians in clinic. It is simpler, safer and cheaper than female sterilization.

Advantages:

1. One time method.
2. Most effective protection against preganancy.
3. Less risk of complications.

Disadvantages:

1. Short-term complications like temporary bruising, infection and bleeding, known as hematoma can occur.
2. Post operative pain syndrome can occur.

(ii) Female sterilization: Female sterilization is the most widely used family planning method in the world and one of the most effective. It can be done by two most common procedure, laparoscopy and minilaparotomy.

Minilaparotomy: *It* involves a small abdominal incision through which a surgeon usually lifts the fallopian tubes out of the abdomen to block them. The incision is 2-5 cm above the pubic hairline when a woman has not recently been pregnant or 1.5-3 cm just below the navel or umbilicus for postpartum procedures. This procedure is appropriate for women during interval, post-abortion and immediate postpartum periods. During interval minilaparotomy, the provider may use a uterine elevator, a metal instrument which is inserted into the vagina to raise the uterus. This makes it easier to move the pelvic structures so that the tubes are near the incision site.

Laparoscopy: It uses a laparoscope, a narrow lighted tube through which a surgeon is able to see into the abdominal cavity and pelvic structure. This optical instrument is inserted through a small puncture near the navel, or umbilicus. The same opening, or sometimes a second puncture, is used to manipulate the organs and block the tubes. It is recommended only for women in the interval period or following first-trimester abortion (when gestation is less than 12 weeks). Laparoscopy should not be performed on women during the postpartum period because of the orientation and the vascular nature of the postpartum uterus.

Once a month pill: A contraceptive tablet that acts like the morning-after pill but could be taken up to a month after sex is probably scientifically possible and would be welcomed by women, scientists have said.

Male pill:

A reversible format of hormonal birth control for men under development, which consists of progestin plus a soupcon of testosterone injected every 34 months to stop sperm production.

Some men use withdrawal to try to prevent pregnancy, when they pull their penis out of their partner's vagina before ejaculating. However, this is not a recommended method of contraception. Sperm can be released from the penis before ejaculation.

Pregnancy test:

A pregnancy test attempts to determine whether a woman is pregnant. Markers that indicate pregnancy are found in urine and blood, and pregnancy tests require sampling one of these substances. The first of these markers to be discovered, human chorionic gonadotropin (hCG), was discovered in 1930 to be produced by the syncytiotrophoblast cells of the fertilised ova (eggs). While hCG is a reliable marker of pregnancy, it cannot be detected until after implantation. This results in false negatives if the test is performed during the very early stages of pregnancy. HCG can be detected via blood 8 days after fertilization of the egg, and in the urine 10 days after. Obstetric ultrasonography may also be used to detect pregnancy. Obstetric ultrasonography was first practiced in the 1960s; the first home test kit for hCG was invented in 1968. The kits went on the market in the United States and Europe in the mid-1970s.

Modern test:

The test for pregnancy which can give the quickest result after fertilization is a rosette inhibition assay for early pregnancy factor (EPF). EPF can be detected in blood within 48 hours of fertilization. However, testing for EPF is expensive and time-consuming.

Most chemical tests for pregnancy look for the presence of the beta subunit of hCG, or human chorionic gonadotropin, in the blood or urine. hCG can be detected in urine or blood after implantation, which occurs six to twelve days after fertilization. Quantitative blood (serum beta) tests can detect hCG levels as low as 1 mIU/mL, while urine test strips have published detection thresholds of 10 mIU/mL to 100 mIU/mL, depending on the brand. Qualitative blood tests generally have a threshold of 25 mIU/mL, and so are less sensitive than some available home pregnancy tests. Most home pregnancy tests are based on lateral-flow technology.

With obstetric ultrasonography the gestational sac sometimes can be visualized as early as four and a half weeks of gestation (approximately two and a half weeks after ovulation) and the yolk sac at about five weeks' gestation. The embryo can be observed and measured by about five and a half weeks. The heartbeat may be seen as early as six weeks, and is usually visible by seven weeks' gestation.

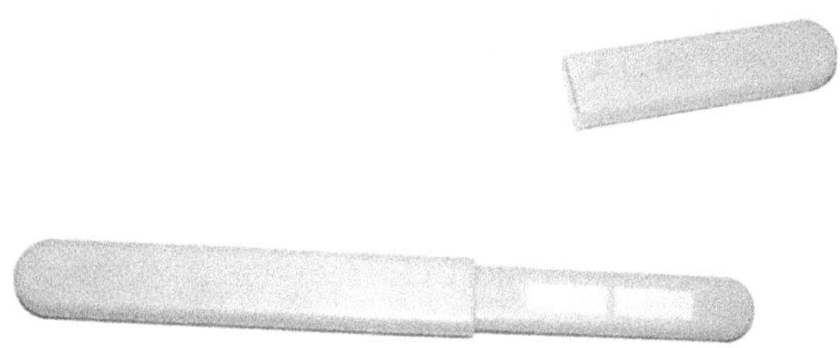

Fig. 17.5: A modern pregnancy test

Accuracy:

A systematic review published in 1998 showed that home pregnancy test kits, when used by experienced technicians, are almost as accurate as professional laboratory testing (97.4%). When used by consumers, however, the accuracy fell to 75%: the review authors noted that many users misunderstood or failed to follow the instructions included in the kits. Improper usage may cause both false negatives and false positives.

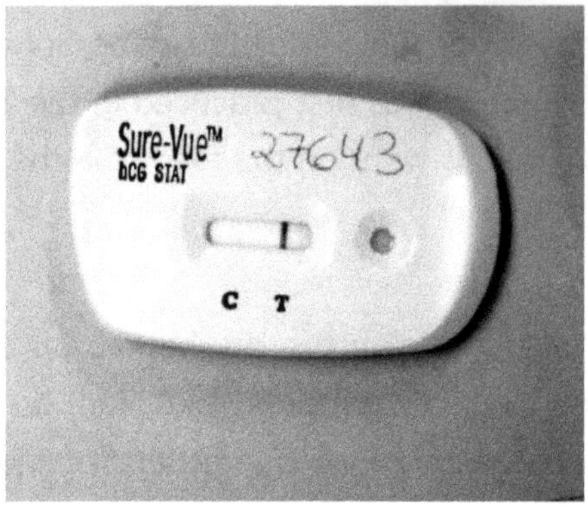

Fig. 17.6: The control line of this pregnancy test is blank, making the test invalid

Timing of test:

False negative readings can occur when testing is done too early. Quantitative blood tests and the most sensitive urine tests usually begin to detect hCG shortly after implantation, which can occur anywhere from 6 to 12 days after ovulation. hCG levels continue to rise through the first 20 weeks of pregnancy, so the chances of false negative test results diminish with time (gestation age). Less sensitive urine tests and qualitative blood tests may not detect pregnancy until three or four days after implantation. Menstruation occurs on average 14 days after ovulation, so the likelihood of a false negative is low once a menstrual period is late.

Ovulation may not occur at a predictable time in the menstrual cycle, however. A number of factors may cause an unexpectedly early or late ovulation, even for women with a history of regular menstrual cycles. Using ovulation predictor kits (OPKs), or charting the fertility signs of cervical mucus or basal body temperature give a more accurate idea of when to test than day-counting alone.

The accuracy of a pregnancy test is most closely related to the day of ovulation, not of the act of intercourse or insemination that caused the pregnancy. It is normal for sperm to live up to five days in the fallopian tubes, waiting for ovulation to occur. It could take up to 12 further days for implantation to occur, meaning even the most sensitive pregnancy tests may give false negatives up to 17 days after the act that caused the pregnancy. Because some home pregnancy tests have high hCG detection thresholds (up to 100 mIU/mL), it may take an additional three or four days for hCG to rise to levels detectable by these tests — meaning false negatives may occur up to three weeks after the act of intercourse or insemination that causes pregnancy.

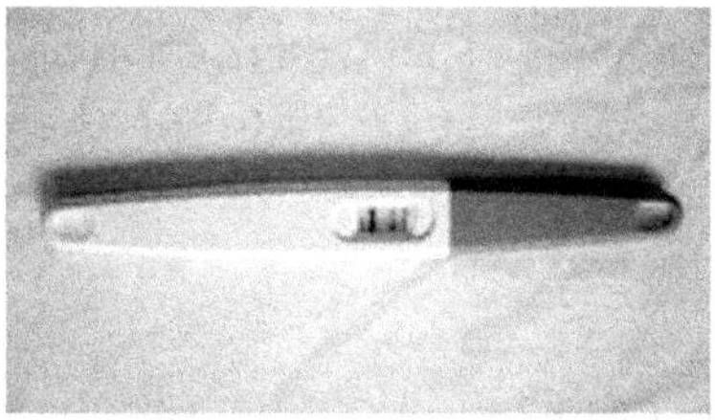

Fig. 17.7: The control line on the left of this pregnancy test is visible, suggesting that the test result is valid. A pale purple line has also appeared on the right hand side (the test line) which clearly signifies that the woman is pregnant

False positives:

False positive test results may occur for several reasons, including errors of test application, use of drugs containing the hCG molecule, and non-pregnant production of the hCG molecule. Urine tests can be falsely positive in those that are taking the medications: chlorpromazine, phenothiazines and methadone among others.

Spurious evaporation lines may appear on many home pregnancy tests if read after the suggested 3–5 minute window or reaction time, independent of an actual pregnancy. False positives may also appear on tests used past their expiration date.

A woman who has been given an hCG injection as part of infertility treatment will test positive on pregnancy tests that assay hCG, regardless of her actual pregnancy status. However, some infertility drugs (e.g., clomid) do not contain the hCG hormone.

Some diseases of the liver, cancers, and other medical conditions may produce elevated hCG and thus cause a false positive pregnancy test. These include choriocarcinoma and other germ cell tumors, IgA deficiencies, heterophile antibodies, enterocystoplasties, gestational trophoblastic diseases (GTD), and gestational trophoblastic neoplasms.

Viability:

Pregnancy tests may be used to determine the viability of a pregnancy. Serial quantitative blood tests may be done, usually 3–4 days apart. Below an hCG level of 1,200 mIU/ml the hCG usually doubles every 48–72 hours, though a rise of 50–60% is still considered normal. Between 1,200 and 6,000 mIU/ml serum the hCG usually takes 72–90 hours to double, and above 6,000 mIU/ml, the hCG often takes more than four days to double. Failure to increase normally may indicate an increased risk of miscarriage or a possible ectopic pregnancy.

Ultrasound is also a common tool for determining viability. A lower than expected heart rate or missed development milestones may indicate a problem with the pregnancy. Diagnosis should not be made from a single ultrasound, however. Inaccurate estimations of fetal age and inaccuracies inherent in ultrasonic examination may cause a scan to be interpreted negatively. If results from the first ultrasound scan indicate a problem, repeating the scan 7–10 days later is reasonable practice.

Diagnostic Tests during Pregnancy:

Diagnostic tests are tests that involve taking a sample of the placenta, the amniotic fluid, or fetal blood. The samples are then sent away and examined in a laboratory for chromosomal or genetic abnormalities. The two main diagnostic tests are amniocentesis and chorionic villus sampling, or CVS. Since both of these tests carry a small risk of miscarriage, you will need to carefully consider the advantages and disadvantages of the tests before going ahead with either of them.

First Trimester Prenatal Screening Tests:

First trimester screening is a combination of fetal ultrasound and maternal blood testing performed during the first trimester of pregnancy. This screening process can help to determine the risk of the fetus having certain birth defects. Screening tests may be used alone or in combination with other tests.

There are three parts of first trimester screening:

- **Ultrasound test for fetal nuchal translucency (NT):** Nuchal translucency screening uses an ultrasound test to examine the area at the back of the fetal neck for increased fluid or thickening.
- **Two maternal serum (blood) tests:** The blood tests measure two substances found in the blood of all pregnant women:
- **Pregnancy-associated plasma protein screening (PAPP-A):** A protein produced by the placenta in early pregnancy. Abnormal levels are associated with an increased risk for chromosome abnormality.
- **Human chorionic gonadotropin (hCG):** A hormone produced by the placenta in early pregnancy. Abnormal levels are associated with an increased risk for chromosome abnormality.

  When used together as first trimester screening tests, nuchal translucency screening and maternal blood tests have a greater ability to determine if the fetus might have a birth defect, such as Down syndrome (trisomy 21) and trisomy 18.

  If the results of these first trimester screening tests are abnormal, genetic counseling is recommended. Additional testing such as chorionic villus sampling, amniocentesis, cell-free fetal DNA, or other ultrasounds may be needed for accurate diagnosis.

Second Trimester Prenatal Screening Tests:

Second trimester prenatal screening may include several blood tests, called multiple markers. These markers provide information about a woman's risk of having a baby with certain genetic conditions or birth defects. Screening is usually performed by taking a sample of the mother's blood between the 15th and 20th weeks of pregnancy (16th to 18th is ideal). The multiple markers include:

- **Alpha-fetoprotein screening (AFP):** This blood test measures the level of alpha-fetoprotein in the mothers' blood during pregnancy. AFP is a protein normally produced by the fetal liver and is present in the fluid surrounding the fetus (amniotic fluid), and crosses the placenta into the mother's blood. The AFP blood test is also called MSAFP (maternal serum AFP).

  Abnormal levels of AFP may signal the following:

  - Open neural tube defects (ONTD), such as spina bifida.
  - Down syndrome.
  - Other chromosomal abnormalities.

- Defects in the abdominal wall of the fetus.
- Twins--more than one fetus is making the protein.
- A miscalculated due date, as the levels vary throughout pregnancy.

- **hCG:** This is human chorionic gonadotropin hormone (a hormone produced by the placenta).
- **Estriol:** This is a hormone produced by the placenta.
- **Inhibin:** This is a hormone produced by the placenta.

Chorionic villi sampling (CVS):

Chorionic villi are fragments of placental tissue. Because the placenta originates from the fertilized egg, the chromosomes in the cells that make up the placenta are representative of your baby's chromosomes. During CVS, a small amount of tissue from your placenta is removed and tested in a laboratory to reveal if your baby has a chromosomal disorder such as Down syndrome or another trisomy disorder, such as trisomy 18. CVS is done between 10 and 12 $^{1}/_{2}$ weeks' gestation and the results are usually available within 7 to 10 days. The procedure can also definitely identify your baby's sex, if you want to know. If you don't want to have this information, make your wishes clear before the test. In rare cases, the doctor will be unable to perform CVS due to the placenta's position. In this case, you may be asked to return for an amniocentesis at 15 weeks.

Amniocentesis:

This is the most common diagnostic test, done at around 15 to 19 weeks of pregnancy. The amniotic fluid around your baby mainly consists of your baby's urine and contains cells from your baby's skin and urinary tract. During amniocentesis, a number of cells are collected from the amniotic fluid. They are then sent to a laboratory and grown in a cell culture, until there is a sufficient number of cells to examine your baby's chromosomes and identify whether your baby has a chromosomal abnormality such as Down syndrome. Amniotic fluid can also be tested for high levels of the substance alpha-fetoprotein (AFP), which could mean that your baby has a neural tube defect such as spina bifida or anencephaly. Other DNA testing can also be done during amniocentesis to check for congenital conditions that may run in either parent's family.

Questions

1. Define family planning.
2. Write the objectives of family planning.
3. Enlist the various methods of family planning
4. Write the advantages and disadvantages of oral pills
5. Explain the method of terminal sterilization in males.
6. Explain the method of terminal sterilization in females.
7. Explain the spacing method of family planning.
8. Explain the advantages and disadvantages of barrier method.

***

Experiment No. 18

Aim: To find out total red blood cells (RBCs) count in human blood.

Apparatus and material:

1. Compound Microscope with mechanical stage and oil immersion lens
2. Neubauer slide
3. Disposable pricking needle
4. Bulb pipette for RBCs count

Material:

1. 70% alcohol
2. Distilled water
3. RBC diluting fluid
4. Cotton

Principle:

Since the normal RBC count runs in millions, the count is made possible by diluting the sample of blood before counting and subsequently multiplying the count by the dilution factor.

Composition of RBC diluting fluid (Haymes solution):

Sodium chloride 0.5 g	To maintain isotonicity of the fluid, therefore RBCs remain suspended in the solution
Sodium sulphate 2.5 g	To prevent aggregation of the RBCs
Mercuric chloride 0.25g	Preservative, antibacterial, antifungal
Distilled water 100 ml	Solvent

Theory:

Erythrocytes (Red Blood Cells):

These are circular biconcave non-nucleated discs with a diameter of about 7 microns. Measurements of red cell numbers, volume and haemoglobin content are routine and useful assessments made in clinical practice. The symbols in brackets are the abbreviations commonly used in laboratory reports.

Erythrocyte count: This is the number of erythrocytes per litre (1) or per cubic millimetre (mm^3) of blood.

Packed cell volume or haematocrit (PCV): This is the volume of red cells in 1 litre or 1 mm^3 of whole blood.

Mean cell volume (MCV): This is the average volume of cells, measured in femtolitres (fl = 101-15 litre).

Haemoglobin (Hb): This is the weight of haemoglobin in whole blood, measured in grams per 100 ml.

Mean cell haemoglobin (MCH): This is the average amount of haemoglobin in each cell, measured in pictograms (pg = 101-12 gram).

Mean cell haemoglobin concentration (MCHC): This is the amount of haemoglobin in 100 ml of red cells.

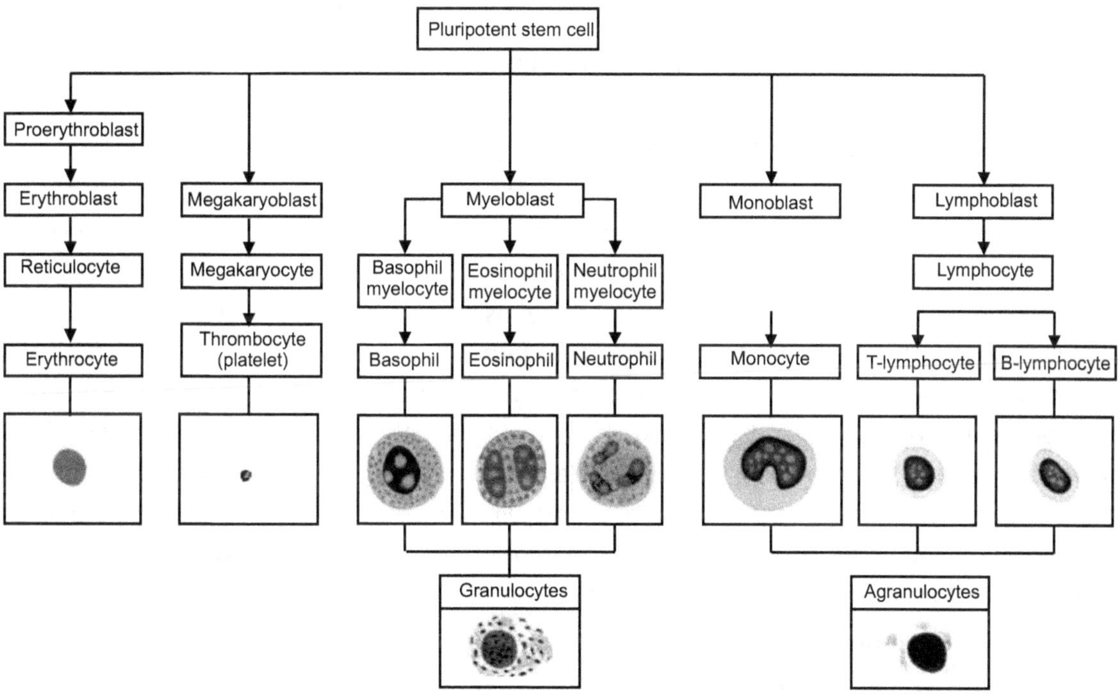

Fig. 18.1: Haemopoiesis: Stages in the development of blood cells

Development and life span of erythrocytes: Erythrocytes are formed in red bone marrow, which is present in the ends of long bones and in flat and irregular bones. They pass through several stages of development before entering the blood. Their life span in the circulation is about 120 days. The process of development of red blood cells from pluripotent stem cells takes about 7 days and is called erythropoiesis shown in Fig. 18.1. It is characterised by two main features:

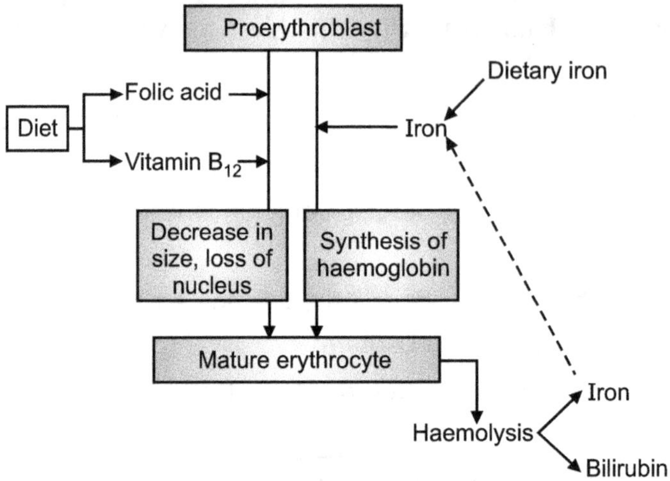

Fig. 18.2: Maturation of the cell

Maturation of the cell: During this process the cell decreases in size and loses its nucleus. These changes depend on a number of factors, especially the presence of Vitamin B_{12} and folic acid. These are present in sufficient quantity in a normal diet containing dairy products, meat and green vegetables. If the diet contains more than is needed, they are stored in the liver. Absorption of Vitamin B_{12} depends on a glycoprotein called intrinsic factor secreted by parietal cells in the gastric glands. Together they form the intrinsic factor-vitamin Bu complex (IF-B_{12}). During its passage through the intestine, the bound vitamin is protected from enzymatic digestion, and is absorbed in the terminal ileum. The effects of deficient intake of vitamin B_{12} do not appear for several years because there are large stores in the liver. Folic acid is absorbed in the duodenum and jejunum where it undergoes change before entering the blood. Signs of deficiency are apparent within a few months. Deficiency of either vitamin B_{12} or folic acid leads to impaired red cell production.

Formation of haemoglobin inside the cell:

Formation of haemoglobin: Haemoglobin is a complex protein, consisting of *globin* and an iron-containing substance called haem, and is synthesised inside developing erythrocytes in red bone marrow. Haemoglobin in mature erythrocytes combines with oxygen to form oxyhaemoglobin, giving arterial blood its characteristic red colour. In this way the bulk of oxygen absorbed from the lungs is transported around the body to maintain a continuous oxygen supply to all cells. Haemoglobin is also involved, to a lesser extent, in the transport of carbon dioxide from the body cells to the lungs for excretion. Each haemoglobin molecule contains four atoms of iron. Each atom can carry one molecule of oxygen; therefore one haemoglobin molecule can carry up to four molecules of oxygen. Haemoglobin is said to be saturated when all its available binding sites for oxygen are filled. When oxygen levels are low, only partial saturation is possible.

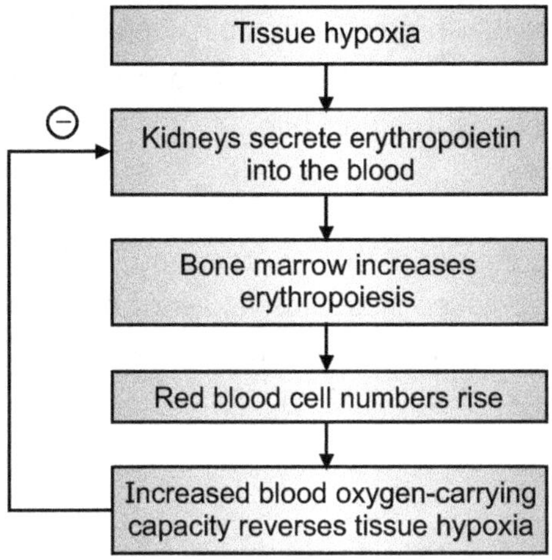

Fig. 18.3: Control of erythropoietin

The number of red cells remains fairly constant, which means that the bone marrow produces erythrocytes at the rate at which they are destroyed. This is due to a homeostatic negative feedback mechanism (Fig. 18.3). The primary stimulus to increased erythropoiesis is hypoxia, i.e. deficient oxygen supply to body cells. This occurs when:

- The oxygen-carrying power of blood is reduced by e.g. haemorrhage or excessive erythrocyte breakdown (haemolysis) due to disease.
- The oxygen tension in the air is reduced, as at high altitudes. Hypoxia increases erythrocyte formation by stimulating the production of the hormone erythropoietin, mainly by the kidneys. Erythropoietin stimulates an increase in the production of proerythroblasts and the release of increased numbers of reticulocytes into the blood. These changes increase the oxygen-carrying capacity of the blood and reverse tissue hypoxia, the original stimulus. When the tissue hypoxia is overcome, erythropoietin production declines (Fig. 18.3). When erythropoietin levels are low, red cell formation does not take place even in the presence of hypoxia, and anaemia (the inability of the blood to carry adequate oxygen for body needs) develops. It is believed that erythropoietin regulates normal red cell replacement, i.e. in the absence of hypoxia.

Destruction of erythrocytes:

The life span of erythrocytes is about 120 days and their breakdown, or haemolysis, is carried out by phagocytic reticuloendothelial cells. These cells are found in many tissues but the main sites of haemolysis are the spleen, bone marrow and liver. As erythrocytes age, changes in their cell membranes make them more susceptible to haemolysis. Iron released by haemolysis is retained in the body and reused in the bone marrow to form haemoglobin (Fig. 18.2). Biliverdin is formed from the protein part of the erythrocytes. It is almost completely reduced to the yellow pigment bilirubin, before it is bound to plasma globulin and transported to the liver. In the liver it is changed from a fat-soluble to a water-soluble form before it is excreted as a constituent of bile.

Determination of RBC indices:

Principle:

The values for RBC count, Haemoglobin content and packed cell volume can be used to obtain certain RBC indices also called Absolute values of blood index. These indices indicate the size and haemoglobin concentration within the RBC and thus help in diagnosing the type of anaemia. The various indices are given as under:

Mean corpuscular volume: Volume of a single RBC in cubic microns. It can be derived from the formula as:

$$MCV\ (\mu m^3) = \frac{\text{PCV per 100 ml blood}}{\text{RBC count in million per cumm}} \times 10$$

Normal range 78-94 μm^3

1. RBCs with normal MCV are called **Normocytes.**
2. RBCs whose MCV exceed normal range are **Macrocytes.**
3. RBCs with MCv below normal range are **Microcytes.**

Mean corpuscular haemoglobin: Average amount of haemoglobin in a single RBC in pictogram or micro-micro gram. It can be derived from the formula as:

MCH (pg) = Haemoglobin in gm%/RBC count in million per cumm × 10

Normal range = 28-32 pg

Mean corpuscular haemoglobin concentration: Amount of haemoglobin expressed as percentage of the volume of a RBC or it is the haemoglobin concentration in a single RBC.

$$MCHC = \frac{\text{Haemoglobin in gm\%}}{\text{PCV per 100 ml blood}} \times 100$$

Normal range = 32%-38%.

1. If the MCHC is within normal range, the RBC is **Normochromic.**
2. If the MCHC value is below normal range, the RBC is **Hypochromic**. This usually indicate that an individual is suffering from iron deficiency.
3. MCHC values never exceed 38% because RBCs can not hold haemoglobin beyond its saturation point i.e. metabolic limit of the cells haemoglobin forming mechanism therefore anaemic can never be hyperchromic.

Procedure:

1. See that apparatus is clean at hand.
2. Examine the counting chamber under microscope and confirm that it is clean and the ruled lines clearly seen.
3. Pour about 2 ml of RBC diluting fluid in watch glass. Hold the RBC pipette mouth piece between the infolded lips and the pipette to hang down.
4. Prick the finger and suck the blood in pipette.
5. Fill the pipette with blood accurately without the entry of air bubble up to mark 0.5. If any air bubble enters in the pipette discard it by tapping on a dry adsorbent cotton plug.

6. Dip the tip of pipette in the RBC diluting fluid in the watch glass and suck accurately up to the 101 mark.
7. Hold the pipette horizontally and fold rubber tubing and roll it between the palms of hands to mix thoroughly with RBC diluting fluid.
8. Clean the counting chamber and cover slip.
9. Place the counting chamber on a plane horizontal and on vibration free surface. It can be charged even on the microscope stage.
10. Place the covers slip resting over the flanges on both side of the depressed platform.
11. Roll the pipette to ensure complete mixing of cells in fluid immediately before charging.
12. Blow out at least three drops of fluid. Note that the stem fills up with one part of only diluting fluid and contains no blood at all. It is necessary to remove this fluid before charging.
13. Watch the size of drop as it comes out.
14. Hold the pipette at an angle of about 45 degree and touch it in the center of depressed platform and edge of cover glass while fluid obtaining down and a drop is being formed. As surface of drop is formed it will touch the inner edges of slide and cover glass by the capillary action. The drop of blood mixture spread uniformly without the air bubble.
15. The fluid run down in a more or if any air bubble is left on the slide, remove cover slip. Clean the slide. Replace it and charge it again.
16. After charging the counting chamber correctly, allow the fluid to settle for a period of 2 to 3 min on the stage of microscope before actual counting starts. The counting cannot be undertaken when the cells are moving their position due to current in the fluid.
17. Fix the slid on the stage of the compound microscope with the clips. Allow to settle the cells for 2 min.
18. Focus the R1 section of 16 squares under the low power.
19. Change over to high power 45 × Focus and adjust the light till you see the cells and rolling clearly.
20. Move the slide carefully till you bring of 16 smallest squares under visual field.
21. Start counting the cells in right upper and left small square.
22. The cells lying across the upper horizontal and left vertical border line should be counted in the square under consideration. While those lying across the lower horizon and right vertical border line should be counted in the adjacent square.
23. First count the cells in the upper 4 horizontal square. From left to right then drop down and count the cells in the second row towards the left. Now drop down and count the cells in the 3 towards the right and so on till you count the cells in all the squares i.e. R2.
24. Count the cells as previously in this big block.

25. Similarly count the cells in the lower right R3, left right R4, and center block R5.
26. In any case the counting should not be undertaken if preparation has dried.

Observation table:

R_1

R_2

R_5

R_3

R_4

Calculations:

Dilution correction factor:

We have diluted 0.5 part of blood in 100 parts of solution (blood + diluting fluid)

Dilution is 0.5 to 100

i.e. 1 to 200

so dilution correction factor is 200.

Volume correction factor:

Each R section has an area of 0.04 sq.mm and depth of 0.1 mm.

Area of 1 R section × Depth of 1 R section = Volume of 1 R section

$$0.04 \text{ sq.mm} \times 0.1 \text{ mm} = 0.004 \text{ cumm.}$$

$$\text{Total volume of 5 R sections} = \text{Volume of 1R section} \times \text{Number of R sections}$$

$$= 0.04 \times 5$$

$$= 0.02 \text{ cu mm}$$

$$\text{Volume Correction Factor} = \frac{\text{Volume desired}}{\text{Volume used}}$$

$$= \frac{1.00 \text{ cu mm}}{0.02 \text{ cu mm}}$$

$$\text{Volume Correction Factor} = 50$$

Now total red blood cell count can be calculated as follows

Number of cells in 5R sections × Dilution factor × Volume Correction Factor × 200 × 50

Result:

Total RBC count in my blood = Million in per cubic mm.

Normal RBCs count

In male: 5 to 6.5 million in per cubic mm.

In Female: 4 to 5.5 million in per cubic mm.

Polycythemia vera: Increase in the RBC count.

Objectives:

1. To understand neubauers chamber layout for RBC and dimensions count.
2. To indentify RBC.
3. To understand the ability in uniform spreading of the blood film over the squares.
4. To understand the ability in proper charging of squares.
5. To understand the calculation from observation of the number of RBC's.

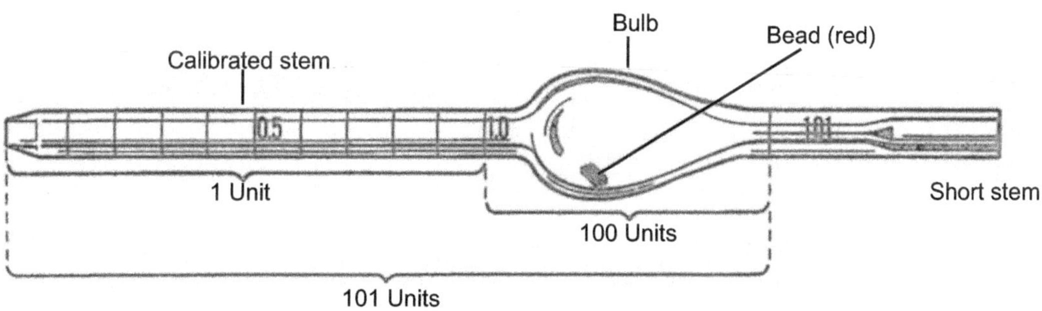

Fig. 18.4: Buble pipette for RBC's count

Questions

1. What are RBCs? Write their functions.
2. Define Erythropoiesis.
3. What is normal count of RBC in men, women and infants?
4. Justify the statement "RBC count is more in men than women".
5. Write the composition of RBC diluting fluids.
6. Write significance of determination of RBC count.
7. What is haemolysis?
8. Enlist the physiological and pathological conditions in which RBC count increases.

***

Experiment No. 19

Aim: To find out total white blood cells (WBCs) count in human blood.

Apparatus and material:

1. Compound Microscope with mechanical stage and oil immersion lens
2. Neubauers Slide
3. Sterile disposable pricking needle
4. Bulb pipette for WBCs count

Material:

1. 70% alcohol.
2. Distilled water.
3. WBC diluting fluid.

Principle:

Since the normal WBC count runs in millions, the count is made possible by diluting the sample of blood before counting and subsequently multiplying the count by the dilution factor. WBC count is much lower than the RBC count, much lesser dilution (1 : 20) is employed.

Composition of WBC diluting fluid or Turks solution:

Glacial acetic acid - 3 ml. To lyse or destroy the membrane of WBCs, RBCs, Platelets.

Gention violet 1% aqueous solution - 1 ml. To stain the nuclei of WBCs deep.

Violet black so that they can be identified easily.

Distilled water - 100 ml. To make 100 ml.

Theory:

Leukocytes (white blood cells):

These cells have an important function in defending the body against microbes and other foreign materials. Leukocytes are the largest blood cells and they account for about 1% of the blood volume. They contain nuclei and some have granules in their cytoplasm. There are two main types:

(a) Granulocytes (polymorphonuclear leukocytes)
   - neutrophils, eosinophils and basophils

(b) Agranulocytes
   - monocytes and lymphocytes.

(a) Granulocytes (polymorphonuclear leukocytes):

During their formation, granulopoiesis, they follow a common line of development through myeloblast to myelocyte before differentiating into the three types (Fig 19.1). All granulocytes have multilobed nuclei in their cytoplasm. Their names represent the dyes they take up when stained in the laboratory. Eosinophils take up the red acid dye, eosin; basophils take up alkaline methylene blue; and neutrophils are purple because they take up both dyes.

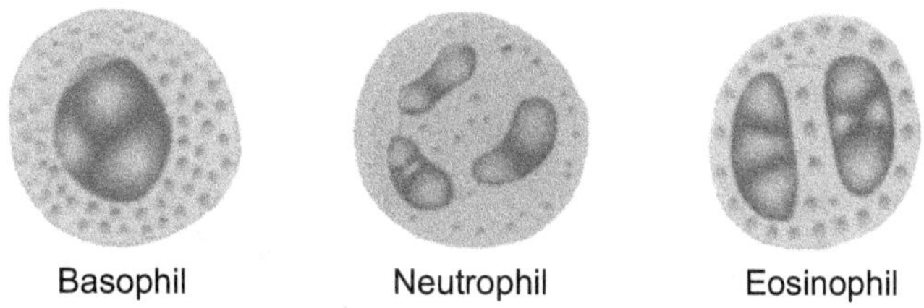

Fig. 19.1: The granulocytes (granular leukocytes)

Neutrophils:

Their main function is to protect against any foreign material that gains entry to the body mainly microbes, and to remove waste materials, e.g. cell debris. They are attracted in large numbers to any area of infection by chemical substances, released by damaged cells, called chemotaxins.

Neutrophils pass through the capillary walls in the affected area by amoeboid movement (Fig. 19.2).

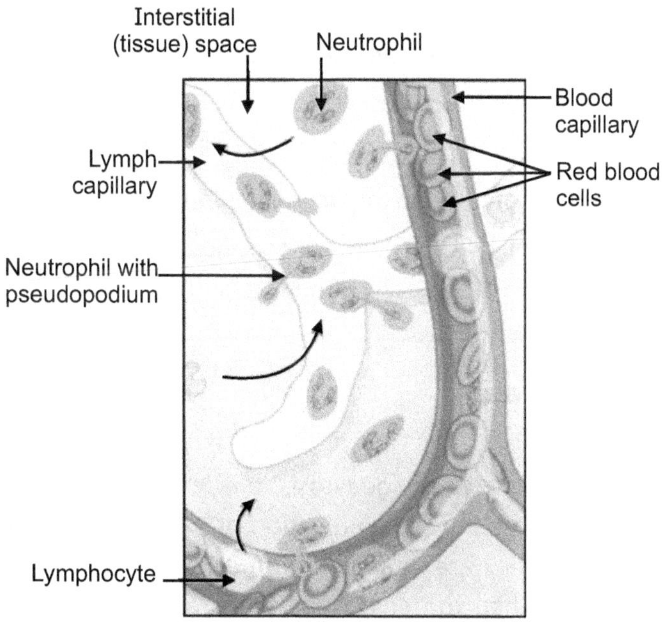

Fig. 19.2: Amoeboid movement of leukocytes

There after they engulf and kill the microbes by phagocytosis (Fig. 19.3). Their granules are lysosomes that contain enzymes that digest the engulfed material. The pus that may form in the affected area consists of dead tissue cells, dead and lives microbes, and phagocytes killed by microbes. There is a physiological increase in circulating neutrophils following strenuous exercise and in the later stages of normal pregnancy.

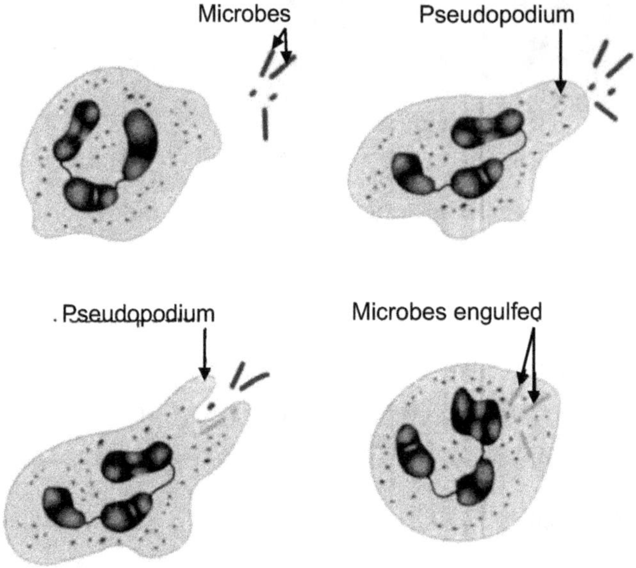

Fig. 19.3: Phagocytic action of Neutrophils

Numbers are also increased in:

- Microbial infection.
- Tissue damage, e.g. inflammation, myocardial infarction, burns, crushes injuries.
- Metabolic disorders, e.g. diabetic ketoacidosis, acute Gout.
- Leukaemia.
- Heavy smoking.
- Use of oral contraceptives.

Eosinophils:

Eosinophils, although capable of phagocytosis, are less active in this than neutrophils; their specialised role appears to be in the elimination of parasites, such as worms, which are too big to be phagocytosed. They are equipped with certain toxic chemicals, stored in their granules, which they release when the eosinophil binds an infecting organism. Eosinophils are often found at sites of allergic inflammation, such as the asthmatic airway and skin allergies. There, they promote tissue inflammation by releasing their array of toxic chemicals, but they may also dampen down the inflammatory process through the release of other chemicals, such as an enzyme that breaks down histamine.

Basophils:

Basophils, which are closely associated with allergic reactions, contain cytoplasmic granules packed with heparin (an anticoagulant), histamine (an inflammatory agent) and other substances that promote inflammation. Usually the stimulus that causes basophils to release the contents of their granules is an allergen (an antigen that causes allergy) of some type. This binds to antibody-type receptors on the basophil membrane. A cell type very similar to basophils, except that it is found in the tissues, not in the circulation, is the mast cell. Mast cells release their granule contents within seconds of binding an allergen, which accounts for the rapid onset of allergic symptoms following exposure to, for example, pollen in hay fever.

(b) Agranulocytes:

The types of leukocyte with a large nucleus and no granules in their cytoplasm are monocytes and lymphocytes and they make up 25% to 50% of all leukocytes (Fig. 19.4).

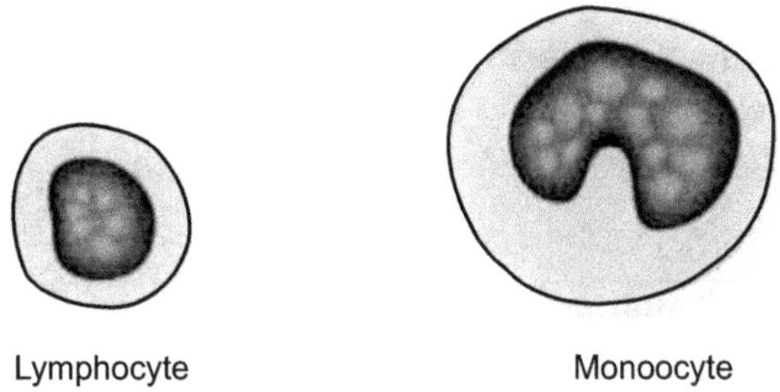

Fig. 19.4: Agranulocytes

The Agranulocytes Monocytes:

These are large mononuclear cells that originate in red bone marrow. Some circulate in the blood and are actively motile and phagocytic while others migrate into the tissues where they develop into macrophages. Both types of cell produce interleukin 1 which:

- Acts on the hypothalamus, causing the rise in body temperature associated with microbial infections.
- Stimulates the production of some globulins by the liver.
- Enhances the production of activated T-lymphocytes. Macrophages have important functions in inflammation and immunity.

The Monocyte-Macrophage System:

This system, which is sometimes called the reticuloendothelial system, consists of the body's complement of monocytes and macrophages. Some macrophages are mobile whereas others are fixed. These include:

- Histiocytes in connective tissues.
- Microglia in the brain.
- Kupffer cells in the liver.
- Alveolar macrophages in the lungs.
- Sinus-lining macrophages (reticular cells) in the spleen, lymph nodes and thymus gland.
- Mesangial cells in the glomerulus of nephrons in the kidney.
- Osteoclasts in bone.

Macrophages function in close association with monocytes in the blood and with lymphocytes which influence their activity. They are actively phagocytic and if they encounter large amounts of foreign or waste material, they tend to multiply at the site and 'wall off the area, isolating the material, e.g. in the lungs when foreign material has been inhaled. Their numbers are increased in microbial infections, collagen diseases and some noninfective bowel conditions.

Lymphocytes:

Lymphocytes are smaller than monocytes and have large nuclei. They circulate in the blood and are present in great numbers in lymphatic tissue such as lymph nodes and the spleen. Lymphocytes develop from pluripotent stem cells in red bone marrow, and then travel in the blood to lymphoid tissue elsewhere in the body where they are activated, i.e. they become immunocompetent which means they are able to respond to antigens (foreign material). Examples of antigens include:

- Cells regarded by lymphocytes as abnormal, e.g. those that have been invaded by viruses, cancer cells, tissue transplant cells.
- Pollen from flowers and plants.
- Fungi.
- Bacteria.
- Some large molecule drugs, e.g. penicillin, aspirin.

Although all lymphocytes originate from one type of stem cell, when they are activated in lymphatic tissue, two distinct types of lymphocyte are produced T-lymphocytes and B-lymphocytes.

Procedure:

1. See that apparatus is clean at hand.
2. Examine the counting chamber under microscope and confirm that it is clean and you are able to see the ruled lines clearly.
3. Pour about 2 ml of WBC diluting fluid in watch glass. Hold the wbc pipette mouth piece between the infolded lips and the pipette to hang down.
4. Prick the finger and suck the blood in pipette.
5. Fill the pipette with blood accurately without the entry of air bubble up to mark 0.5. If any air bubble enters in the pipette discard it by tapping on a dry adsorbent cotton plug.
6. Dip the tip of pipette in the WBC diluting fluid in the watch glass and suck accurately up to the 11 mark.
7. Hold the pipette horizontally and fold rubber tubing and roll it between the palms of hands to mix thoroughly with WBC diluting fluid.

8. Clean the counting chamber and cover slip.
9. Place the counting chamber on a plane horizontal surface and on vibration free. It can be charged even on the microscope stage.
10. Place the covers slip resting over the flanges on both side of the depressed platform.
11. Roll the pipette to ensure complete mixing of cells in fluid immediately before charging.
12. Blow out at least three drops of fluid. Note that the stem fills up with one part of only diluting fluid and contains no blood at all. It is necessary to remove this fluid before charging.
13. Watch the size of drop as it comes out.
14. Hold the pipette at an angle of about 45 degree and touch it in the center of depressed platform and edge of cover glass while fluid obtaining down and a drop is being formed as surface of drop is formed will touch the inner edges of slide and cover glass by the capillary action. The drop of blood mixture spread uniformly without the air bubble.
15. The fluid run down in a more or if any air bubble is left on the slide, remove cover slip. Clean the slide. Replace it and charge it again.
16. After charging the counting chamber correctly, allow the fluid to settle for a period of 2 to 3 min on the stage of microscope before actual counting starts. The counting can not be undertaken when the cells are moving their position due to current in the fluid.
17. Fix the slide on the stage of the compound microscope with the clips. Allow to settle the cells for 2 min.
18. Focus the large corner square under the low power 10X objective.
19. Change over to high power and adjust the light till you see the cells and rolling clearly.
20. Move the slide carefully till you bring of 16 smallest squares under visual field.
21. Start counting the cells in right upper corner large squares, right lower large corner square, left upper corner square, left lower large square. And in this way count cells from 64 smallest squares.
22. While counting the cells lying across the upper horizontal and left vertical border line should be counted in the square under consideration. While those lying across the lower horizontal and right vertical border line should be counted in the adjacent square.
23. First count the cells in the upper 4 horizontal square from left to right then drop down and count the cells in the second row towards the left. Now drop down and count the cells in the 3 row towards the right and so on till you count the cells in all 16 smallest squares and note down reading of each dried preparation.

Observation table:

W_1

W_2

W_4

W_3

Calculations:

Dilution correction factor:

We have diluted 0.5 part of blood in 10 parts of solution (blood + diluting fluid)

Dilution is 0.5 to 10i.e 1 to 20

So dilution correction factor is 20.

Volume correction factor:

Each W section has an area of 1 sq.mm and depth of 0.1 mm.

Area of 1 W section × Depth of 1 W section = Volume of 1 W section

1sq.mm × 0.1 mm = 0.1 cumm.

Total volume of 4 W sections = Volume of 1 W section × Number of W sections

= 0.1 × 4

= 0.4 cu mm.

Volume Correction Factor = Volume desired/Volume used

= 1.00 cu mm/0.4 cu mm

Volume Correction Factor = 2.5

Now total red blood cell count can be calculated as follows:

Number of cells in 5R sections × Dilution factor × Volume Correction Factor

× 2.5 × 20

Result:

Total WBC count in my blood = per cubic mm.

(Normal WBCs count – 4000-10000/cu mm of blood.)

Conclusion:

Total leukocyte count of the sample is ...... (normal/abnormal) showing presence of leukocytosis /leukocytopenia.

Leukocytosis: WBC count is increased.

Leukocytopenia: WBC count is less.

Objective:

1. To understand Neubauers chamber layout for WBC and dimensions count.
2. To indentify WBC.
3. To understand the ability in uniform spreading of the blood film over the squares.
4. To understand the ability in proper charging of squares.
5. To understand the calculation from observation the no. of WBC's.

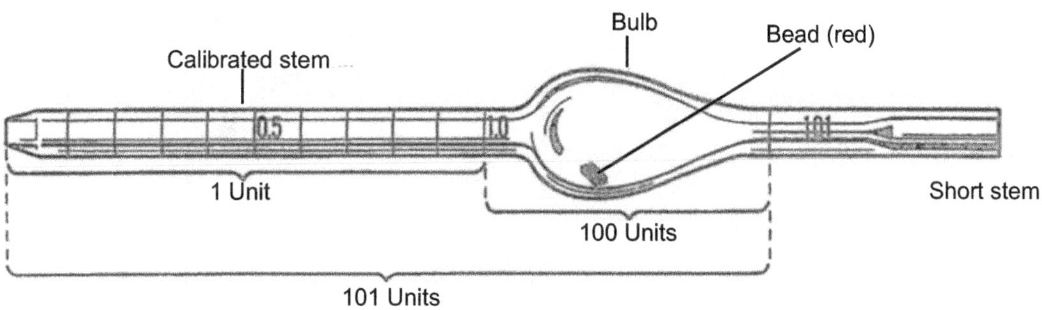

Fig. 19.5: Buble pipette for RBC's count

Questions

1. Give composition of WBC diluting fluid.
2. What is dilution of blood during total WBC count?
3. Sate any 4 physiological conditions and causes of Leukocytosis.
4. What is leukemia? What are its types?
5. Where the leucocytes are formed?
6. Give the formation of granulocytes.
7. What is dilution factor in WBC count
8. Why gentian violet is used in WBC diluting fluid?
9. Why glacial acetic acid is used in WBC diluting fluid?
10. What is leucopenia. Enlist physiological condition and causes of leucopenia.

***

Experiment No. 20

Aim: To study permanent slide of gonads.

Introduction:

For Pathological and biological research, the specimen usually undergoes a complex histological preparation that involves fixing it to prevent decay, removing any water contained in it, replacing the water with paraffin, cutting it into very thin sections using a microtome, placing the sections on a microscope slide, staining the tissue using various stains to reveal specific tissue component, clearing the tissue to render it transparent and covering it with a coverslip and mounting medium.

Especially useful for educational purposes and for those who do not want to undertake the labourious process of creating slides, prepared microscope slides are available in all areas of science, including biology like plant, animal and single-cell organism.

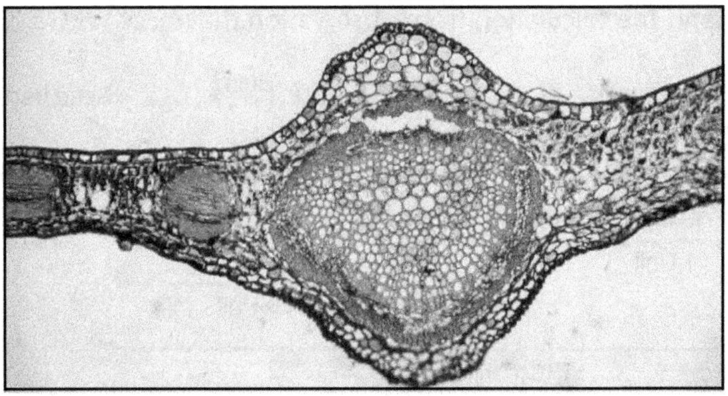

Fig. 20.1: Example of Stating of Toluidine Blue

Microscope slide preparation:

Usually three under mentioned techniques are used for the purpose

Jeffrey's Method:

1. Take the dried or fresh plant material and make very thin slices of it. Boil the material in water by keeping it in a test-tube. After sometime when the material becomes air free and settles down in the bottom of the test tube, it is macerated in a solution.
2. The maceration solution may be prepared as follows:
   (i) 10% Nitric acid (i.e., 90 ml water + 10 ml nitric acid).
   (ii) 10% Chromic acid (i.e., 90 ml water + 10 ml chromic acid).
   Mix (i) and (ii) acids.
3. Now take the material in this maceration solution in a test tube. Heat this solution and separate the material in small pieces by piercing a needle to the material. Stop heating as soon as the material becomes soft and pulp like.

4. Now transfer this pulpy material to a watch glass. Drain out all the maceration fluid. Wash the material several times with water so that the acid traces are removed completely. Now strain the material with aqueous safranin and mount it in glycerine or glycerine jelly. The material may also be passed through alcohol series for making permanent slides.

Harlow's Method:

Treat the slice and boiled material with chlorine water for two hours. Now wash the material with water. After proper washing boil the water in sodium sulphite for fifteen minutes. Now transfer this fluid to a watch glass. Drain out the water. Tease the material with the help of a needle for the separation of tissues. Prepare temporary or permanent mounts.

Schultze's Method:

Make thin slices of the material and boil it in water in a test tube. Now fill the test tube with concentrated nitric acid, and add a few crystals of potassium chlorate to it. Heat it gently till material becomes white. Now transfer the fluid through the watch glass and drain out the liquid leaving material alone. Wash the material with water. Tease the material with the help of a needle, so that the cells may be separated from each other. Stain the material and make temporary or permanent mounts.

Staining:

The tissue differentiation is possible only by staining the different tissues with different stains. The stains are the chemical dyes having different reactions with the cell wall of the tissue and thus giving a particular stain to a particular tissue. For example, the acid dye stains unlignified tissue while the basic ones stain lignified tissue.

Single Staining:

The plant materials having no differentiation of tissues (e.g. Algae, fungi, bryophytes) are stained by this process.

Double Staining:

The plant material having highly differentiated tissues (e.g. Pteridophyta, gymnosperms, angiosperms, etc.) are stained by this process. Double staining involves the use of two dyes, one acidic and other basic. The acidic dye stains unlignified tissues while the basic one stains lignified tissues. Some important dyes are as follows:

1. Safranin:

Alcoholic		
Sr. No.	**Ingredients**	**Quantity**
1.	Safranin	1 gm
2.	Alcohol 95%	50 c.c.
3.	Distilled water	50 c.c

Aqueous		
Sr. No.	**Ingredients**	**Quantity**
1.	Safranin	1 gm
2.	Distilled water This is mainly used to stain lignified tissues	10 c.c.
3.	Distilled water	10 c.c.

2. Crystal violet or Gentian violet:

Sr. No.	Ingredients	Quantity
1.	Crystal violet	1 gm
2.	Distilled water It is basic violet dye and stains lignified tissues.	100 c.c.

3. Aniline Blue:

Sr. No.	Ingredients	Quantity
1.	Aniline Blue	1 gm
2.	Alcohol (95%) of	
3.	Distilled water It stains cellulose walls.	100 c.c.

4. Erythrosine:

Sr. No.	Ingredients	Quantity
1.	Erythrosine	1 gm
2.	Absolute Alcohol	5 c.c.
3.	Clove oil It is used to stain gelatinous sheath e.g. Algae.	95 c.c.

5. Eosin:

Sr. No.	Ingredients	Quantity
1.	Eosin	1 gm
2.	Water It stains cytoplasm.	100 c.c.

6. Light Green:

Sr. No.	Ingredients	Quantity
1.	Light Green	1 gm
2.	Alcohol 95%	2.5 c.c.
3.	Clove oil - It is used to stain cellulose and lignified cell walls.	95 c.c

7. Fast Green:

Sr. No.	Ingredients	Quantity
1.	Fast Green	0.5 gm
2.	Alcohol 95%	2.5 c.c.
3.	Clove oil	75 c.c.

8. Cotton Blue:

Sr. No.	Ingredients	Quantity
1.	Aniline Blue	0.1 gm
2.	Phenol	25 gm
3.	Glycerine	25 c.c.
4.	Lactic acid	25 c.c.
5.	Distilled water This is used for staining various fungi.	25 c.c.

9. Basic Fuchsin:

Solution A		
Sr. No.	**Ingredients**	**Quantity**
1.	Basic Fuchsin	0.3 gm
2.	Alcohol 95%	10 c.c.
Solution B		
Sr. No.	**Ingredients**	**Quantity**
1.	Phenol (melted)	5 gms
2.	Distilled water	95 c.c.

Mix solution A and B

This is a nuclear stain and also used to stain bacteria.

10. Hematoxylins:

Heidenhain's Hematoxylin		
Sr. No.	**Ingredients**	**Quantity**
1.	Hematoxylin	0.5 gm
2.	Warm distilled water Store in a dark place to ripen at least for four days before use.	100 c.c.

Delafield's Hematoxylin		
Sr. No.	**Ingredients**	**Quantity**
1.	Saturated aqueous solution of ferric ammonium sulphate	100 c.c.
2.	Hematoxylin	1 gm
3.	absolute alcohol	6 c.c.

11. Acetocarmine:

Sr. No.	Ingredients	Quantity
1.	Carmine	1gm
2.	Glacial acetic acid (45%)	100 c.c.

Dissolve 1 gm of carmine in 100 c.c. of boiling 45% acetic acid. Cool this mixture and decant. Add few drops of ferric acetate aqueous solution in the mixture. Cool the mixture abruptly by keeping it in ice. Filter the mixture and stock it in a cool place.

12. Toluidine O: (Toluidine blue O)

Sr. No.	Ingredients	Quantity
1.	Toluidine blue O (C.I. 52040)	0.1 g
2.	Ethanol	sq
3.	Distilled water	100.0 mL

A gonad or sex gland or reproductive gland is a mixed gland that produces the gametes (sex cells) and sex hormones of an organism. In the female species the reproductive cells are the egg cells, and in the male the reproductive cells are the sperm. The male gonad, the testicle, produces sperm in the form of spermatozoa. The female gonad, the ovary, produces egg cells. Both of these gametes, are haploid germ cells.

Regulation:

The gonads are controlled by luteinizing hormone and follicle-stimulating hormone, produced and secreted by gonadotropes in the anterior pituitary gland. This secretion is regulated by gonadotropin-releasing hormone produced in the hypothalamus.

Development of the gonads:

Gonads start developing as a common primordium (an organ in the earliest stage of development), in the form of gonadal ridges, and only later are differentiated to male or female sex organs. The presence of the SRY gene, located on the Y chromosome and encoding the test is determining factor, determines male sexual differentiation. In the absence of the SRY gene from the Y chromosome, the female sex (ovaries instead of testes) will develop. The development of the gonads is a part of the development of the urinary and reproductive organs.

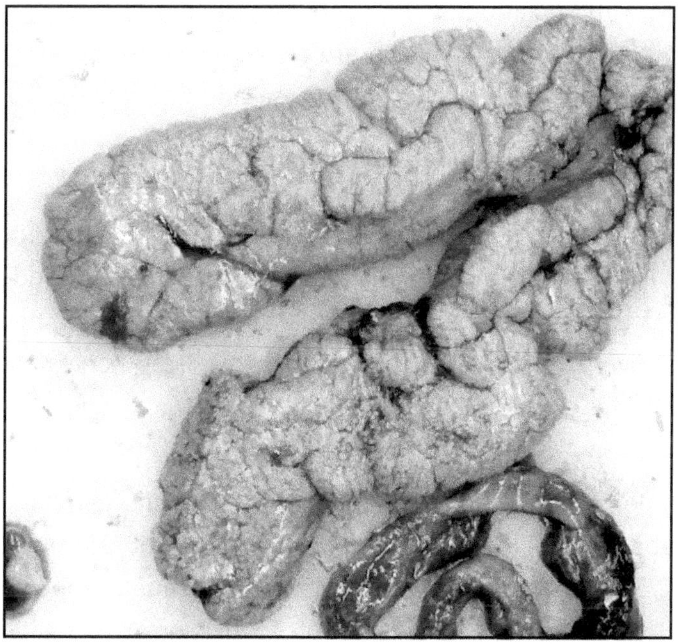

Fig. 20.2: A pair of fresh ovaries of Cyprinus carpio

Questions

1. What is the meaning of permanent slide?
2. Defined Staining.
3. How you prepare permanent slide?
4. Give any one formula of dyes.
5. Comments on regulation of gonads.

***

Experiment No. 21

Aim: To study the histological structure of human slides.

Apparatus:

Permanent glass slides or films of T.S of stomach, small intestine, pancreas, liver, testis, ovary, kidney.

Stomach:

The serosa, or visceral peritoneum, is the outermost layer of the stomach. It consists of an inner layer of connective tissue and an outer layer of simple squamous epithelium. The muscularis of the stomach consist of three layers: an outer longitudinal layer, a middle circular layer, and an inner oblique layer. In some areas of the stomach, such as in the fundus, the three layers blend with one another and cannot be separated. Deep to the muscular layer are the sub mucosa and the mucosa, which are thrown into large folds, called rugae when the stomach is empty. These folds allow the mucosa and sub mucosa to stretch. The folds disappear as the stomach is filled.

Liver:

The liver is covered by a connective tissue capsule and visceral peritoneum, except for the bare area, which is a small area on the diaphragmatic surface surrounded by the coronary ligament. At the porta the connective tissue capsule sends a branching network of septa into the substance of the liver to provide its main support. Vessels, nerves and ducts follow the connective tissue branches throughout the liver.

Small intestine:

The small intestine consists of three parts: the duodenum, jejunum, ileum. The entire small intestine is about 6 m long. The duodenum is about 25 cm long. The jejunum constituting about 2/5 of the total length of the small, intestine is about 2.5 m long and the ileum constituting 3/5 of small intestine, is about 3.5 m long. Two major accessory glands, the liver and the pancreas, are associated with duodenum.

Pancreas:

The pancreas is a complex organ composed of both endocrine and exocrine tissues that perform several functions. The pancreas consists of a head, located within the curvature of duodenum, a body and a tail which extends to the spleen.

Characteristics of epithelial tissue:

The tissue consists of cells arranged in continuous sheets either in single or multiple layers. The cells are closely packed. The intercellular space between the cells is less. The apical surface is the free surface of epithelial cells; it faces the body surface or a body cavity or lumen of internal organ or duct. The free surface may contain cilia or microvilli. The lateral surface of the cells faces adjacent cells on either side. The basal surface adheres to extracellular material such as basement membrane. It has less blood supply. The basement membrane is a thin extracellular layer. It consists of two layers:

(a) The basal lamina,

(b) Reticular lamina

The basal lamina is thin and close to the epithelial cells. It is composted of the epithelial laminin, glycoproteins and proteoglycan. The reticular lamina is closer to underlying connective tissue. It contains fibrous proteins produced by connective tissue cells, i.e., fibroblasts. Function of the basement membrane is to provide point of attachment and support to epithelial cells.

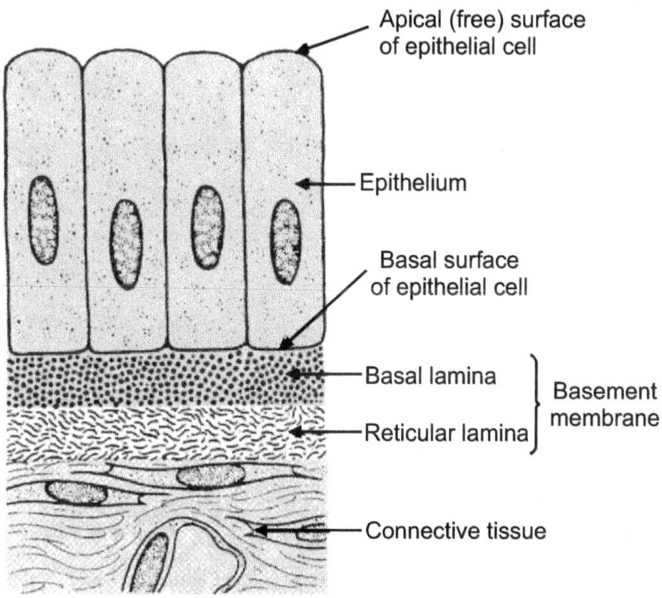

Fig. 21.1: Epithelial tissue

Function:

Epithelial tissue plays many different roles in the body such as :

(1) Protection of underlying tissues – e.g. skin.

(2) Filtration - e.g. in glomerulus.

(3) Secretion - e.g. secretion of mucus.

(4) Absorption - e.g. epithelia in stomach, intestine.

(5) Excretion - e.g. secretory glands.

Two types of epithelial tissue are:

(A) Covering and lining epithelium.

(B) Glandular epithelium.

(A) Covering and Lining Epithelium:

This epithelia forms the outer covering of the skin and some internal organs. It also forms the inner lining of blood vessels, ducts and interior of systems like the digestive, urinary and reproductive systems.

The covering and lining epithelial tissue is further classified according to two characteristics - the arrangement of cells into layers and shape of the cells.

The types of epithelia are:

(I) Simple epithelium:

(a) Simple squamous epithelium

(b) Simple cuboidal epithelium

(c) Simple columnar epithelium

(d) Pseudostratified columner epithelium

(II) Stratified epithelium:

(a) Stratified squamous epithelium

(b) Stratified cuboidal epithelium

(c) Stratified columner epithelium

(d) Transitional epithelium

(I) Simple epithelium:

This consists of a single layer of cells of basement membrane. Tissue functions in diffusion, osmosis, filtration, secretion and absorption.

(a) Simple squamous epithelium:

The squamous cells are the flat thin cells arranged like floor tiles. The simple squamous epithelium consists of a single layer of flat cells. The nucleus is flattened, oval or spherical in shape and centrally located. This tissue appears as a thin sheet.

Endothelium is the simple squamous epithelium lining the heart, blood vessel and lymphatic vessel. Epithelial layer of peritoneum is called as mesothelium.

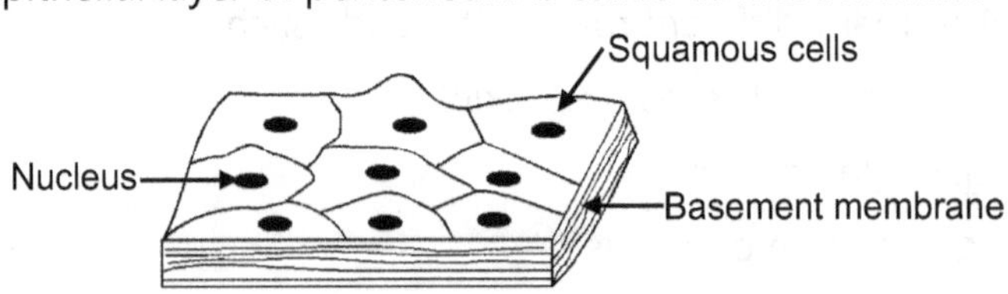

Fig. 21.2: Simple squamous epithelium

Location:

(1) Lining of blood vessel.

(2) Lining of alveoli.

(3) Glomerular capsule in nephron.

Functions:

(1) Filtration.

(2) Diffusion of substances.

(b) Simple cuboidal epithelium:

As the name suggests, the tissue consists of cuboidal shaped cells. The nucleus is usually round and centrally located. The cells are arranged in single layer.

Location:

(1) Thyroid glands, sweat glands and salivary glands.

(2) Lining of ducts of glands and nephron tubules.

(3) Covering of ovaries.

Function:

(1) Secretion

(2) Absorption

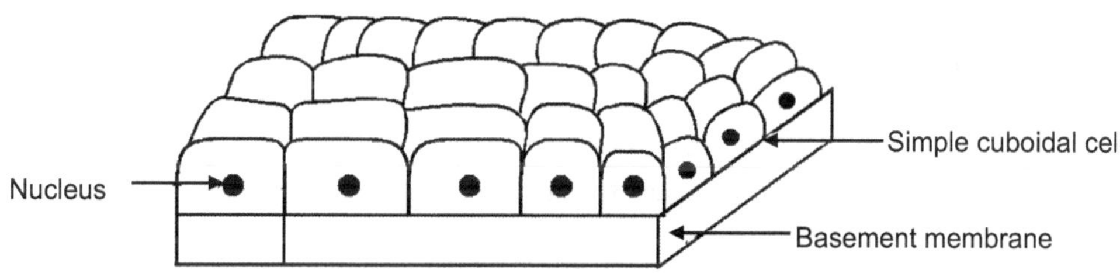

Fig. 21.3: Simple cuboidal epithelium

(c) Simple columnar epithelium:

- The cells in this tissue appear like a column. The nucleus is oval shaped and arranged near the base. Two types of columnar epithelia are non-ciliated columnar epithelium and ciliated columnar epithelium. In the non-ciliated epithelium, the cells do not consist of cells at free apical surface. This epithelium consists of two types of cells - columnar cells with microvilli at apical surface and goblet cells.
- Microvilli are the finger-like projections present in the plasma membrane of cells. These cells increase the surface area of the plasma membrane, e.g. in small intestine, and increase rate of absorption.
- Goblet cells are modified columnar cells that secrete mucus. Mucus is a slightly sticky fluid. The mucus layer acts as lubricant for linings and protects the underlying layer.
- Ciliated columnar epithelium contains the columnar cells that consist of cilia at free apical surface. Cilia are the hair-like processes. The movement of cilia moves fluid, or particles, along the tube.

Location:

(1) Lining of digestive system.
(2) Lining of respiratory system.
(3) Lining of reproductive system.

Function:

(1) Protection
(2) Secretion
(3) Absorption

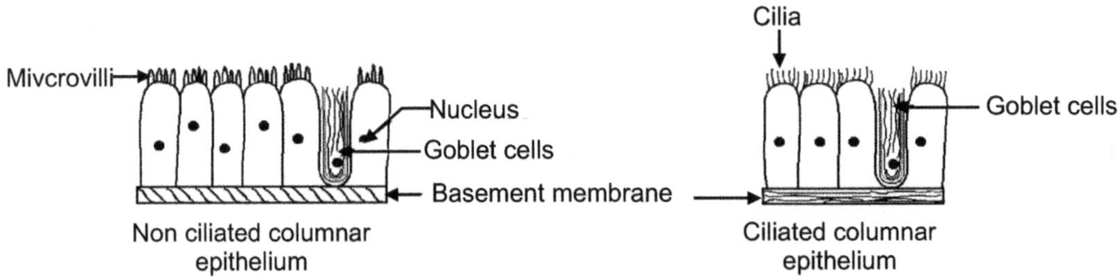

Fig. 21.4: Non ciliated and ciliated columnar epithelium

(d) Pseudostratified columnar epithelium:

The word pseudo means false. The pseudostratified epithelium appears to have multiple layers of cells. The nuclei of the cells lie at different levels and all cells do not reach apical surface.

Location: Airway of upper respiratory tract.

Function: Secretion of mucus and movement of mucus by cilliary action.

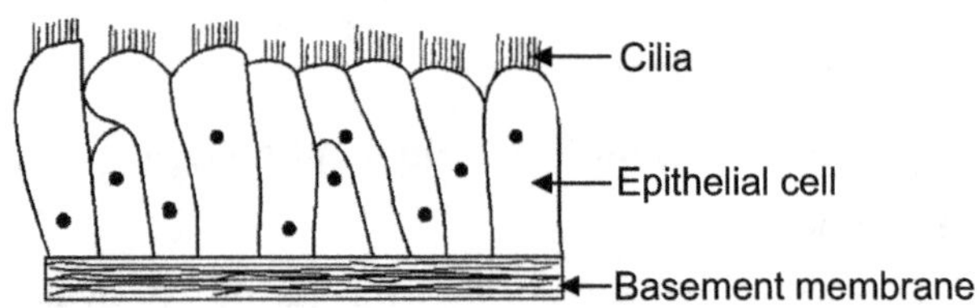

Fig. 21.5: Pseudostratified columnar epithelium

(II) Stratified epithelium:

Stratum means layer. The epithelial tissue consists of two or more layers of cells on basement membrane. This tissue is located at the site of considerable wear and tear, depending upon the shape of apical layer cells.

(a) Stratified squamous epithelium:

The cells of apical layer of this type of epithelium are flat. The cells of deep layers vary in shape from cuboidal to columnar. The basal cells continuously undergo cell division. As new cells grow, the cells of basal layer are pushed upwards and forward, towards the apical layer. As the cells move upward they become dehydrated, shrunken and harder and then die.

Types of stratified squamous epithelium are:

(1) Keratinized squamous epithelium:

The apical layer and underlying several layers of cells are partially dehydrated and contain a layer of keratin. Keratin is a tough fibrous protein that protects the skin and underlying tissue from heat, microbes and chemicals.

Locations: Superficial layer of skin.

Function: Protection.

(2) Non-keratinized squamous epithelium:

Non-keratinized squamous epithelium does not contain keratin in apical layer, or deep layer of cells and remains moist, e.g. lining of mouth and esophagus.

Location:

1. Lining of mouth, esophagus.
2. Part of pharynx.
3. Vagina.

Function: Protection.

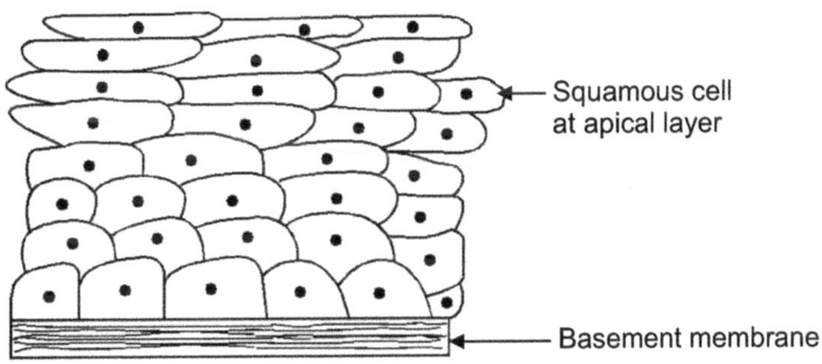

Fig. 21.6: Stratified squamous epithelium

(b) Stratified cuboidal epithelium:

This is a fairly rare type of epithelium. The cells in the apical layers are cuboidal.

Location:

1. Ducts of sweat glands.
2. Ducts of esophageal glands.
3. Part of male urethra.

Function:

(1) Protection
(2) Secretion
(3) Absorption

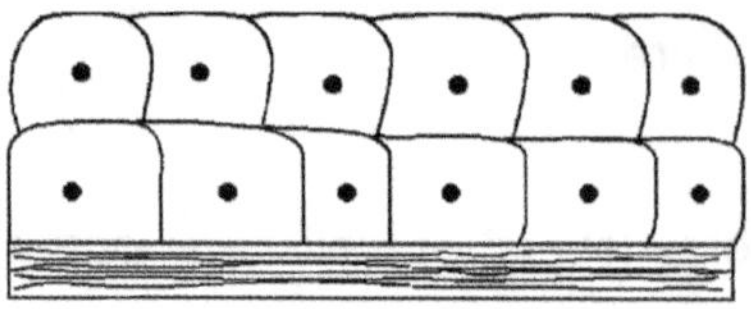

Fig. 21.7: Stratified cuboidal epithelium

(c) Stratified columnar epithelium:

This is also a rare tissue. The cells at the basal layer are usually shortened and irregular in shape and the apical layer cells are columnar in shape.

Location:

(1) Lining of part of urethra.

(2) Excretory ducts of some glands.

(3) Part of the conjunctiva of the eye.

(4) Some esophageal glands.

Function: Protection and secretion.

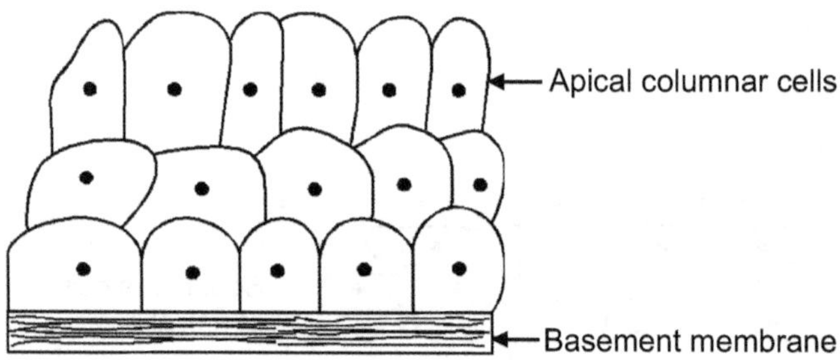

Fig. 21.8: Stratified columnar epithelium

(d) Transitional epithelium:

The tissue has a variable appearance. In its relaxed or unstretched state, the transitional epithelium looks like stratified cuboidal epithelium. Apical layers are large and rounded. As the tissue stretches, the cells become flatter, and appear like stratified squamous epithelium.

Location: lining of urinary bladder; portion of ureter and urethra.

Function: The tissue allows distension of organ to hold variable amount of fluid.

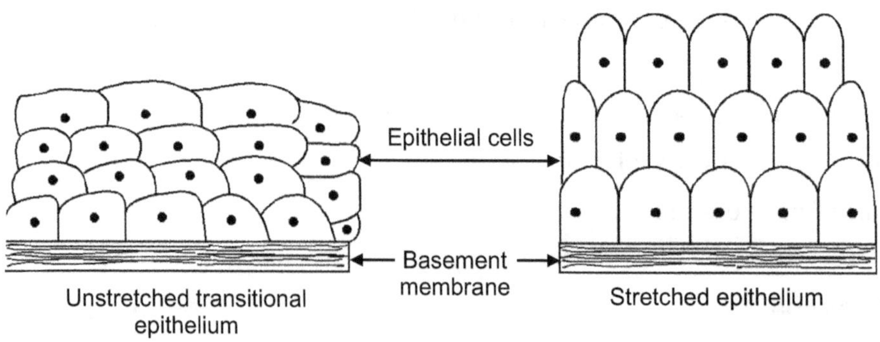

Fig. 21.9: Transitional epithelium

Connective Tissue:

It is the most abundant and widely distributed tissue in the body. It performs various functions. It binds together, supports and strengthens other body tissues. It protects and insulates internal organs. It serves as major transport system in the body. The tissue is also the main source of immune response.

General Characteristics of Connective Tissue:

(1) Connective tissue consists of cells and extracellular matrix. The cells are widely separated from each other in a matrix.

(2) The extracellular matrix consists of protein fibres and ground substance.

(3) The matrix is secreted by immature connective tissue cells. The characteristic cells are fibroblasts, osteoblasts and chondroblasts.

(4) The nature of matrix formed determines the tissue qualities, e.g. in cartilage, it is pliable, while in the bone it is hard and inflexible.

(5) After formation of matrix, the immature cells differentiate and form mature cells. The mature cells are then classified as osteocytes, chondrocytes, etc.

(6) The connective tissue is a highly vascular tissue than epithelium, i.e., it has rich blood supply, cornea of the eye.

Types of connective tissues:

(a) Loose connective tissue.

(b) Dense connective tissue.

(c) Cartilage.

(d) Bone tissue.

(e) Liquid connective tissue.

(a) Loose connective tissue:

The fibres of loose connective tissue are loosely arranged between the cells.

(1) Areolar connective tissue.

(2) Adipose tissue.

(3) Reticular connective tissue.

(1) Areolar connective tissue:

This is the most widely distributed connective tissue. Matrix is semisolid with many fibroblasts widely separated by elastic and collagen fibres.

The cell fibroblasts, macrophages, plasma cells and mast cells are embedded in ground substance.

Location:

(1) Subcutaneous layer deep into the skin.

(2) Supporting blood vessels and nerves.
(3) Between muscles.
(4) In the alimentary canal.
(5) Glands supporting secretary cells.

Function:

1. To provide elasticity and tensile strength.
2. To connect and support other tissues.

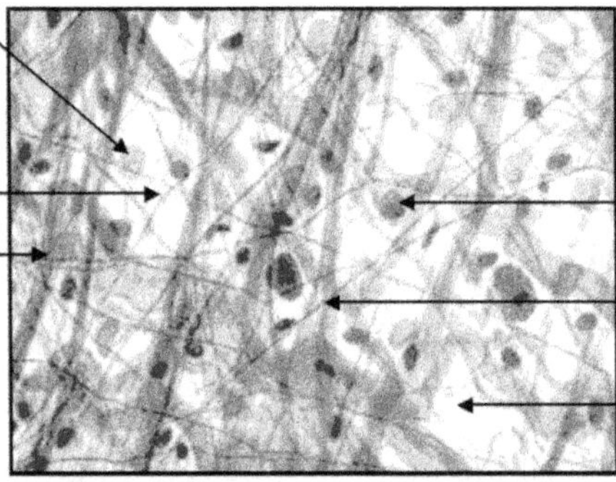

Fig. 21.10: Areolar connective tissue

(2) Adipose tissue:

Adipose tissue consists of fat cells (adipocytes) distributed in a large fat globules in a matrix of areolar tissue. Types of adipose tissue are white adipose and brown adipose.

White adipose tissue:

It constitutes about 20-25 % of body weight. It supports kidneys, eyes, muscle fibres and is also present under the skin, where it acts as thermal insulator.

Brown adipose tissue:

It is present relatively in small amounts, mainly between scapulae, nape of the neck and walls of large blood vessels. It has more extensive capillary network than white adipose tissue. It generates considerable heat and probably helps maintain body temperature in newborns.

Location:

(1) Subcutaneous layer deep into the skin.
(2) Around heart and kidney.
(3) Yellow bone marrow.
(4) Around joints.
(5) Behind eyeball in eye socket.

Function:

(1) Reduces heat loss through skin.
(2) Serves as energy reserve.
(3) Support and protection.
(4) Helps to maintain body temperature.

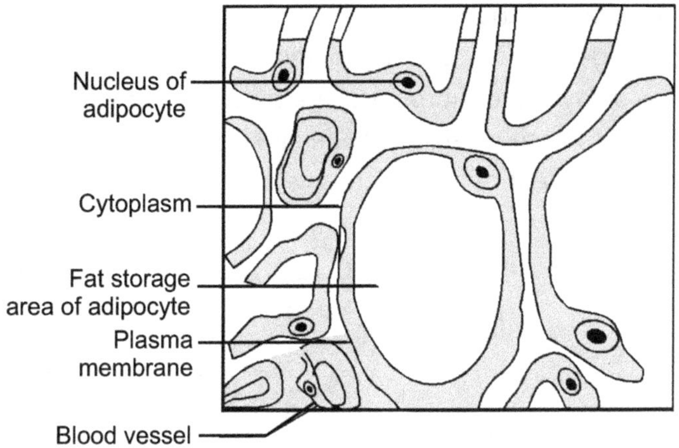

Fig. 21.11: Adipose tissue

(3) Reticular connective tissue:

It consists of interlacing reticular fibres and reticular cells.

Location:

(1) Supporting framework, i.e., stroma of liver, spleen, lymphnodes.
(2) Red bone marrow.
(3) Around the blood vessels and muscles.

Function:

Binds smooth muscle tissue cells, filters and removes worn out blood cells.

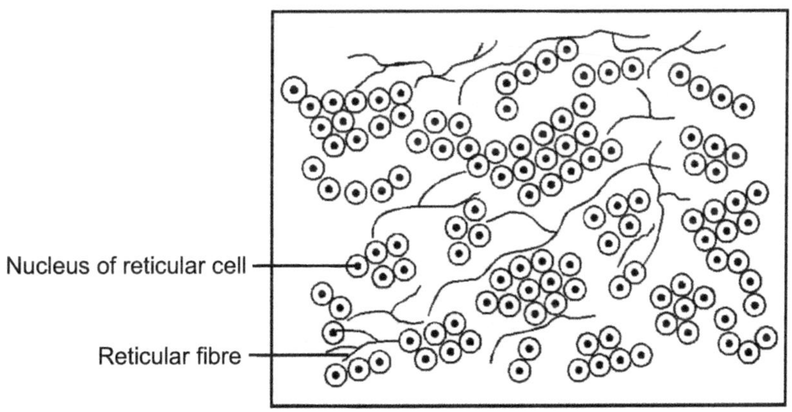

Fig. 21.12: Reticular connective tissue

(b) Dense connective tissue:

This tissue contains of more numerous, thicker and denser fibres. If the number of cells is more, fibres are formed; if they less, than loose connective tissues are formed. The three types of dense connective tissues are:

(1) Dense regular connective tissue.
(2) Dense irregular connective tissue.
(3) Elastic connective tissue.

(1) Dense regular connective tissue:

The bundles of collagen fibres are regularly arranged in a parallel pattern. The extracellular matrix looks shiny white. Fibroblasts are present in rows between bundles.

Location: Tendons, that attach muscle to bone and ligaments that attach bone to bone.

Function: Provides attachment between strong structures.

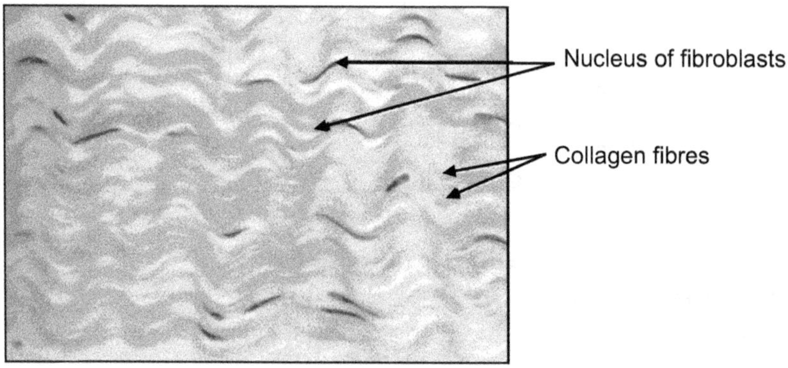

Fig. 21.13: Dense regular connective tissue

(2) Dense irregular connective tissue:

It contains more closely packed collagen fibres. They are usually irregularly arranged and consist of few fibroblasts. The tissue often occurs in sheets, e.g. dermis of skin and pericardium around the heart.

Location:

(1) Form fascia, i.e., tissue beneath skin and around the muscles and organs.

(2) Membrane capsules around various organs.

(3) Pericardium and valves of heart.

Function: It provides strength.

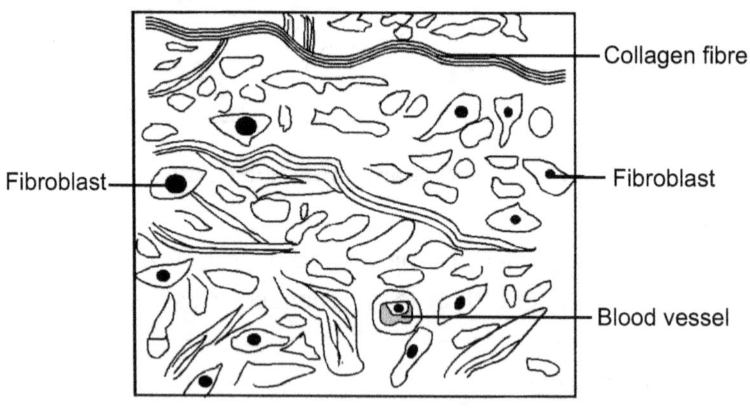

Fig. 21.14: Dense irregular connective tissue

(3) Elastic connective tissue:

The tissue is mainly made up of elastic fibres. The fibroblasts are present in the spaces between the fibres. The elastic tissue is strong and can recoil to its original shape after stretching.

Location:

(1) Lung tissue
(2) Walls of elastic arteries
(3) Trachea
(4) Bronchi
(5) Vocal cords

Function: It allows stretching of various organs.

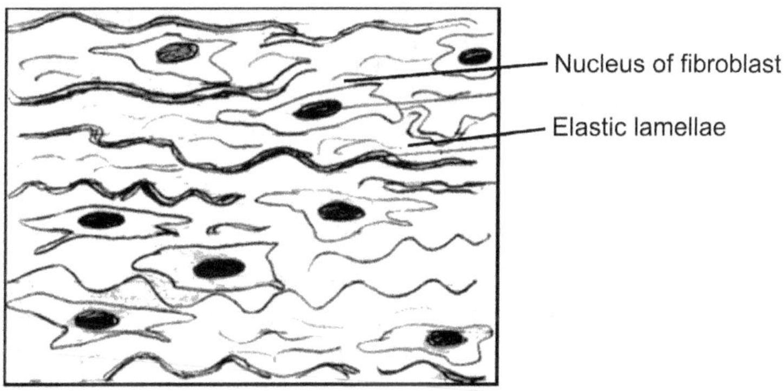

Fig. 21.15: Elastic connective tissue

(c) Cartilage:

Cartilage consists of a dense network of collagen fibres and elastic fibres embedded in gel-like ground substance. The ground substance mainly consists of condroitin sulphate. The cells of mature cartilage are called as chondrocytes. They occur singly or in groups with space called lacunae in extracellular matrix. Perichondrium, a membrane of dense irregular connective tissue, covers the surface of the cartilage. The cartilage has no blood vessels or nerves.

Types of cartilage are:

1. Hyaline cartilage
2. Fibro cartilage
3. Elastic cartilage

1. Hyaline cartilage:

Hyaline cartilage is the most abundant cartilage in the body. It appears as smooth bluish-white tissue. It is weakest of the three types of cartilage. Chondrocytes are found in lacunae in small groups. Matrix is solid and smooth.

Location:

(1) Articulating surfaces of the joints.

(2) Anterior ends of ribs and nose.

(3) Part of larynx, trachea and bronchi.

Function:

(1) Provides smooth surfaces for movements.

(2) Provides flexibility and support.

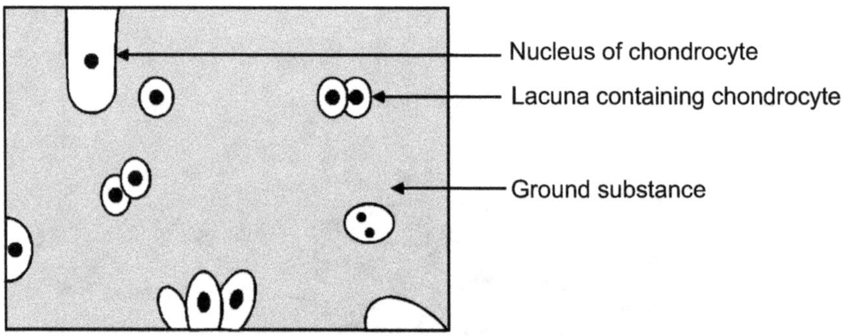

Fig. 21.16: Hyaline cartilage

2. Fibro cartilage:

It is the strongest of the three types of cartilage. It consists of dense masses of white fibres in a matrix. Cells are widely dispersed. It is a tough and slightly flexible tissue.

Location:

(a) The tissue is found as intervertebral disc pads between bodies of vertebras.

(b) Between articulating surface of bones of knee joints.

(c) As ligaments joining bones.

Function:

(1) To provide support.

(2) To help in fusion of tissues.

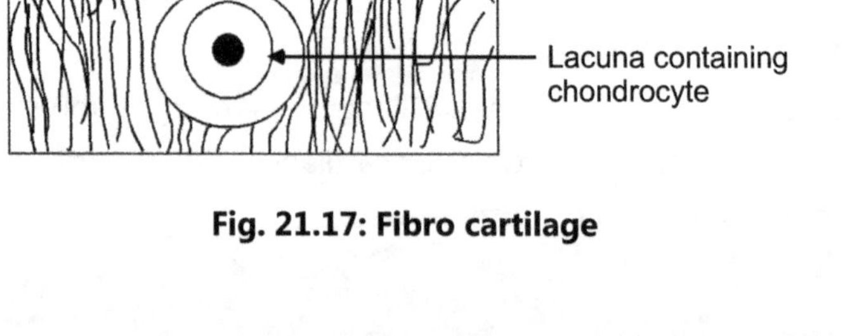

Fig. 21.17: Fibro cartilage

3. Elastic cartilage:

This consists of elastic fibres lying in a solid matrix. The cells are distributed within the fibres. Perichondrium is present in this tissue.

Location: Pinna and lobe of ear.

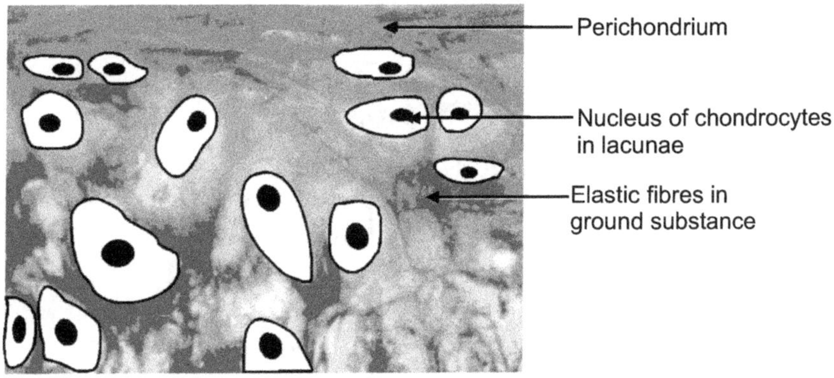

Fig. 21.18: Elastic cartilage

(d) Bone tissue:

Skeletal system consists of cartilage, joints and bones. It supports soft tissues and helps in generating movements. Bones store calcium and phosphorus and house red bone marrow. Bone tissue consists of different connective tissues. Bone tissue is classified either as compact or spongy. Depending on the organization of extracellular matrix and cells. The basic unit of bone tissue is an osteon or haversian system.

Each osteon has four parts:

(1) **Lamellae:** [little plates]: consist of mineral salts (Ca^{++} and phosphates), which are important for bone strength and its hardness.

(2) Lacunae are small spaces between lamellae, which consist of mature bone cells called osteocytes.

(3) Canaliculi are projections from lacunae containing the process of osteocytes. Canaliculi provide routes for nutrients to reach osteocytes and for wastes to leave them.

(4) A central canal contains blood vessels and nerves.

Location: Skeletal system [all bones].

Function:

(1) It provides strength to bones.

(2) It provides hardness to bones.

(3) It is source of calcium and phosphate.

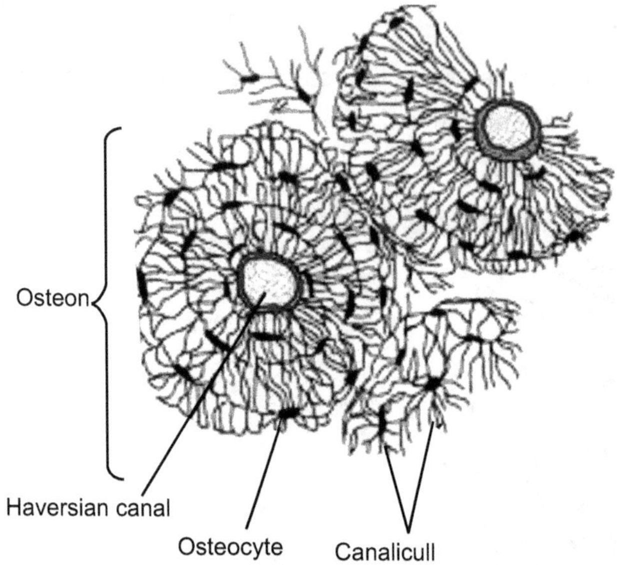

Fig. 21.19: Bone tissue

(e) Liquid connective tissue:

It is divided into two types of tissues:

(1) Blood tissue

(2) Lymph tissue

(1) Blood tissue:

Blood tissue is a connective type of tissue with a liquid extracellular matrix, called blood plasma.

Blood plasma consists of red blood cells, white blood cells and platelets, organic and inorganic substance, dissolved gases, etc.

Location:

Within blood vessels (arteries, arterioles, capillaries, venules and veins) and within chambers of the heart.

Function:

RBCs – For transport of O_2 to body cells and remove CO_2 from them.

WBCs – Involved in phagocytosis, immunity and allergic reactions.

Platelets – Participates in blood clotting.

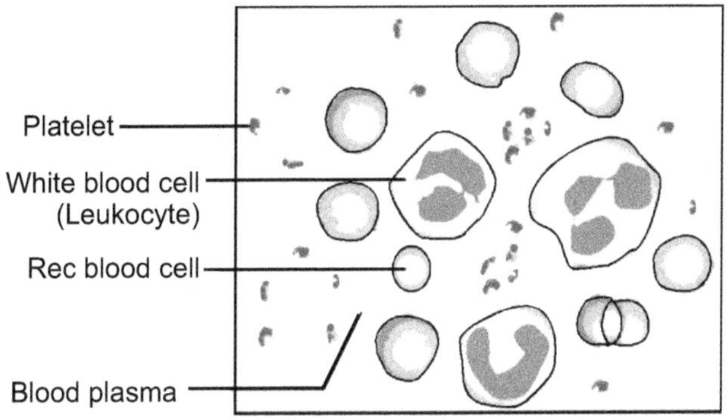

Fig. 21.20: Blood tissue

(2) Lymph tissue:

- Lymph is extracellular fluid that flows in lymphatic vessels.
- It is a connective type of tissue.
- The composition of lymph varies from one part of the body to another.
- It is a specialised form of reticular connective tissue that contains large numbers of lymphocytes.

Location: Lymph vessels.

Function: Drains the ECF from tissues, protection from foreign microorganisms.

Muscular tissue:

Muscular tissue produces body movements, maintains posture and generates heat. It provides protection, to underlining organs.

It is classified into three types:

(1) Skeletal muscle tissue

(2) Cardiac muscle tissue

(3) Smooth muscle tissue

(1) Skeletal muscle tissue:

It is voluntary, as one can contract or relax the tissue by consciously controlling it. Single skeletal muscle fibre is very long, up to 30-40 cm, or about 12-16 inch. Muscle fibre is cylindrical in shape and has nuclei located at the periphery. It contains striations of alternating light and dark bands within the fibres that are visible under light microscope.

Location: It is attached to bones of skeleton.

Function: Motion posture, heat production and protection.

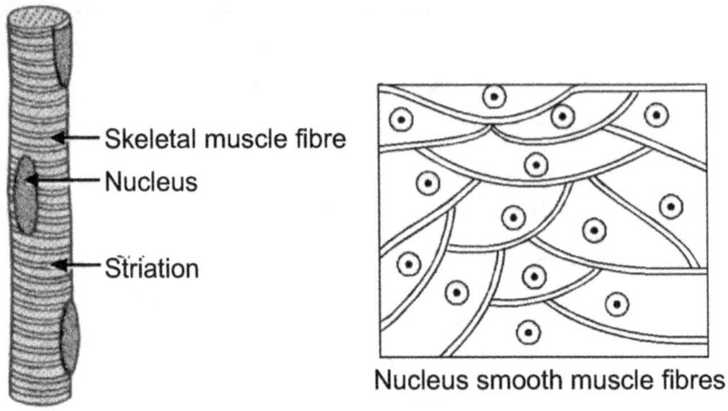

Fig. 21.21: Skeletal muscle tissue

(2) Cardiac muscle tissue:

It forms walls of the heart. It is striated and involuntary. Cardiac muscle fibres are branched and have one centrally located nucleus. They contain intercalated discs.

Location: Heart wall.

Functions: Contacts heart so as to pump blood to all parts of the body.

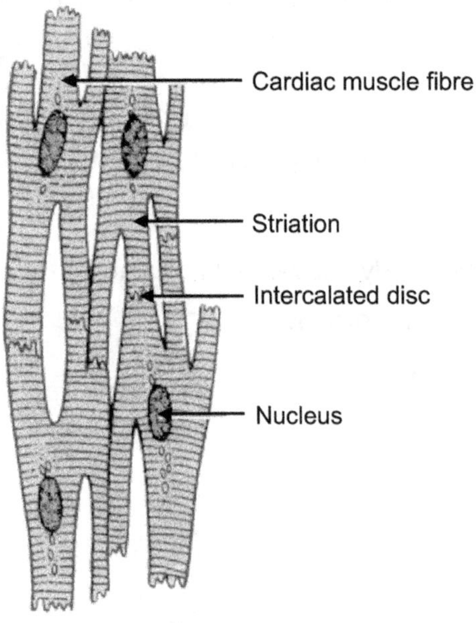

Fig. 21.22: Cardiac muscle tissue

(3) Smooth muscle tissue:

It is located in walls of hollow internal structures such as blood vessels, airways to the lungs, the stomach intestines, gallbladder and urinary bladder.

They are non-striated and involuntary. Smooth muscle fiber is small, thickest in the middle and tapering at each end. It contains single, centrally located, nucleus.

Location: Iris of eye, walls of blood vessels, stomach intestine, uterus, gall bladder etc. airways to lungs.

Functions:

(1) **Motion:** Constriction of blood vessels and airways causes movement of blood and air respectively.

(2) Propulsion of food through gastrointestinal track.

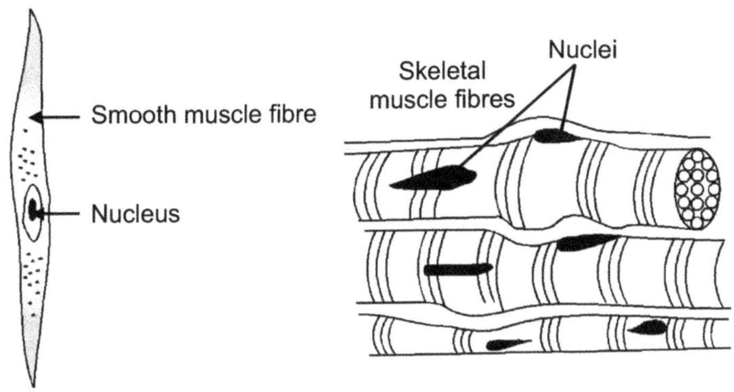

Fig. 21.23: Smooth muscle tissue

Nervous tissue:

It consists of two types of cells:

(1) Neurons

(2) Neuroglia

Neurons convert stimuli into electrical signals called action potential and conduct these signals to other neurons, muscle tissues or glands.

Neurons consist of three basic parts:

(1) Cell body contains nucleus and other organelles.

(2) Dendrites are tapering, highly branched and usually short, cell processes.

(3) Axon is a single, thin cylindrical process that may be very long.

Neuralgias do not generate or conduct nerve impulses. They have important supportive functions. Nervous system consists of vast number of cells called neurones, supported by special types of connective tissues, called neuralgia. Neuron consists of cell body, axon and dendrites. Bundles of axon bound together are called nerves. Neurones are referred to as nerve cells. Nerve cells vary considerably in size and shape.

Axons and dendrites are extensions of cell bodies and form white matter of nervous system. Each nerve axon cell has only one axon, which carries nerve impulses away from the cell body. They are longer than dendrites, as long as 100 cm.

Structure of Axon:

Mebrance of axon is called axolemma. Large axon are surrounded by myclin sheath. This consists of a series of schwann cells arranged along length of axon. Between the layers of plasma membrane fattly substance called myelin is present in myelinated axon while it is absent in non myelinated axons.

Dendrite:

Dendrite is short processes that receive and carry impulse toward cell bodies. They have same structure as axons but are shorter in length.

Location: Nervous system.

Functions:

(1) Sensation of various stimuli.

(2) Converts stimuli into nerve impulse.

(3) Conduct nerve impulse from one neurone to another neurone and effectors cells.

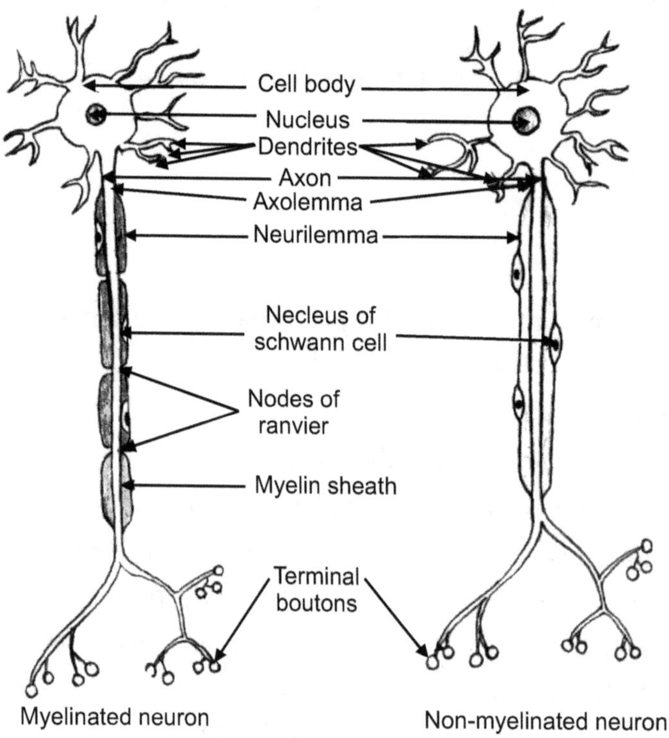

Fig. 21.24: Nervous tissue

(B) Glandular epithelium:

It is formed by cells specialized to produce a fluid secretion. They synthesize, store and secrete extracellular products that are not used by the cell itself but are of importance to other parts of organism. Complex aggregates of glandular epithelial cells parenchyma form the larger multicellular glands or unicellular glands consist of isolated epithelial cells.

It consists of two glands as follow:

(I) Exocrine glands

(II) Endocrine glands

(I) Exocrine glands:

It is maintain connection with the surface epithelium via the tubular ducts through with the secretory product pass to reach the surface.

Histologically it is composed from two parts:

(a) Secretory portion (lat. ***portio secretoria***) contains the cells responsible for the secretory process.

(b) System of ducts (lat. ***ductus glandulae***) transport the secretion to the exterior of the gland.

(II) Endocrine glands:

They are ductless the connection with the surface was obliterated during development and they release their secretory product into the bloodstream.

According to histological structure 3 main types of endocrine glands:

(1) Trabecular

(2) Follicular

(3) Disseminated

1. Trabecular type:

Made from the cords of the cells e.g. adenohypophysis, parathyroid gland, adrenal glands.

2. Follicular type:

The cells form spherical structures e.g. thyroid gland.

3. Disseminated type:

The endocrine cells are placed in groups or separately in another organ e.g. Leydig cells in testis, Langerhans islets of pancreas.

Questions

1. Define tissue.
2. Classify tissue in detail.
3. Explain the characteristics of epithelial tissue.
4. Explain the types of epithelial tissue.
5. Explain the characteristics of muscular tissue.
6. Explain the types of muscular tissue.
7. Explain the characteristics of connective tissue.
8. Explain the types of connective tissue.
9. Explain the characteristics of nervous tissue.
10. Explain the types of nervous tissue.

***

Bachelor of Pharmacy (B. Pharm) course regulations 2014

SEMESTER II

✍ Human Anatomy and Physiology II – Theory	• Dr. S.B. Bhise • Dr. A.V. Yadav
✍ Human Anatomy and Physiology II –Practical	• Md. Rageeb Md. Usman • Dr. Mrunal K. Shirsat • Dr. Jayesh Dwivedi • Dr. Mohammed Zuber Shaikh
✍ Pharmaceutical Organic Chemistry I – Theory	• Dr. K.G. Bothara • Dr. kishor S. Jain • Dr. Pankaj B.Miniyar
✍ Pharmaceutical Organic Chemistry I – Practical	• Dr. Kishor S. Jain • Dr. Pankaj B.Miniyar
✍ Biochemistry – Theory	• Dr. Mrs. P.H. Agarkar
✍ Biochemistry – Practical	• Dr. Mrs. P.H. Agarkar
✍ Pathophysiology – Theory	• Deepa K. Ingawale • Satish K. Mandlik
✍ Environmental sciences – Theory *	• Dr. Kishore Pawar
✍ Computer Applications in Pharmacy – Theory *	• Dhyagude
✍ Computer Applications in Pharmacy – Practical*	
✍ Human Anatomy and Physiology II – Theory	• Prof. (Dr.) Mahesh Prasad • Dr. Antesh Kumar Jha • Mr. Ritesh Kumar Srivastav
✍ Human Anatomy and Physiology II – Practical Practical	• Prof. (Dr.) Mahesh Prasad • Dr. Antesh Kumar Jha • Mr. Ritesh Kumar Srivastav
✍ Pharmaceutical Organic Chemistry I – Theory	• Dr. Abhishek Tiwari • Dr. Neeraj Upmanyu • Anup K. Chakraborty

✍ Pharmaceutical Organic Chemistry I – Practical	• Dr. Abhishek Tiwari • Dr. Mrs. Anita Singh • Dr. Neeraj Upmanyu • Dr. Mrs. Varsha Tiwari
✍ Biochemistry – Theory	• Dr. Sandeep Bansal • Mr. Surya Prakash
✍ Biochemistry – Practical	• Dr. Sandeep Bansal • Mr. Surya Prakash
✍ Pathophysiology – Theory	• Dr. Neeraj Verma • Mr. Sunil Singh • Mr. Santosh Singh Bhadoriya
✍ Environmental sciences – Theory *	• M.K. Gupta • Manish Jaimini • Vikash Pandey
✍ Computer Applications in Pharmacy – Theory *	• Dr. G.D. Gupta • Dr. Shailesh Sharma
✍ Computer Applications in Pharmacy – Practical*	• Dr. G.D. Gupta • Dr. Shailesh Sharma
✍ Human Anatomy and Physiology II – Theory	• Dr. N.B. Sridhara Murthy • Sowmya B.A.
✍ Human Anatomy and Physiology II – Practical Practical	• Dr. N.B. Sridhara Murthy • Sowmya B.A.
✍ Pharmaceutical Organic Chemistry I – Theory	• Dr. Shivakumar Swamy • Bidya Bhushan
✍ Pharmaceutical Organic Chemistry I – Practical	• Dr. Shivakumar Swamy • Bidya Bhushan
✍ Biochemistry – Theory	
✍ Biochemistry – Practical	
✍ Pathophysiology – Theory	
✍ Environmental Sciences – Theory *	• Dr. Kuntal Das
✍ Computer Applications in Pharmacy – Theory *	
✍ Computer Applications in Pharmacy – Practical *	

***

www.ingramcontent.com/pod-product-compliance
Lightning Source LLC
LaVergne TN
LVHW062202171026
850499LV00044B/1834
* 9 7 8 9 3 8 6 9 4 3 5 0 7 *